For Chuck and Michael

Contents

Preface

This book is an interpretation of events in Penny's life as she has told them to me and as I have understood them over the thirteen years of our friendship. It is written in the first person, from Penny's point of view, because midwifery is an intimate business.

I have tried to write her story as accurately as possible, but to protect the privacy of her patients and the Amish community I have changed names and scrambled circumstances. The only names not changed are those of Penny's immediate family members and the names and places in the chapter "Booth." Booth Maternity Hospital, Penny thought, deserves recognition for the quality of its program. Other minor changes in events have been made in the interest of storytelling.

I learned about home birth by assisting at about thirty of them over a period of five years, and I learned about the Amish while living with Penny and her husband in Lancaster County, Pennsylvania, for nearly nine months.

Among the Amish, there is a keen understanding that the work we do is part of the community's work. This book is a result of the work, generosity, insight, and wisdom of many people, but I am especially grateful to Penny and Richard Armstrong, the Bradbury and Howard families, Thelma and Murray Studley, Nancy Nordhoff, Jim Coffin, Lewis O. Saum, Phyllis Hatfield, Don and Lyn Kartiganer, Sue Ellen Loebach, Sue Yates, Lise Wells, Marlene Sanker, and Terry DiJoseph Sears.

Jakes and Lydia Beiler honored me with nothing more and nothing less than their friendship. I hope my appreciation of the Amish people is expressed by this book. I thank each person; knowing them has been an extraordinary privilege.

SHERYL STUDLEY FELDMAN
LANCASTER COUNTY, PENNSYLVANIA
MARCH 1985

The Midwife's Acknowledgments

It has been interesting for me to watch the development of this book: painful, funny, and soul searching in turn. I am a doer, not a recorder, and it has taken me a while to enjoy the thought of publication. I hope this book will help in some small way to ensure the future of the home birth option, and perhaps cause a few readers to pause and reflect on what we lose when we discard the lessons of the past.

I have arrived at this place and acquired and refined my skills with much help and guidance. I wish to acknowledge the people who have taught me the meaning of unconditional love—my parents, Jerry and Arlene Bradbury, and my brothers, Jerry and Bruce; the people who inspired me by their gentle, healing hands and their sense of adventure—Dot Armstrong, R.N., and Ellen Davis, R.N.; the friends who have stayed there through the tough times—Sue Ellen Loebach, Sheryl Feldman, and Rod Potter; the nurse-midwives who provided outstanding examples of skill and caring and who never failed to help and encourage me on my "pioneer" path—Sue Yates, C.N.M., Lois Treize, C.N.M., Shirley Fischer, C.N.M., and Margaret Young.

I am indebted to those conscientious and trusting people who have made the commitment to support me every day—Dr. Trudi Ellenberger and Dr. Mark Cooperstein; and to those who add so much to the quality of the care I am able to give—Shirley Wenger, L.P.N., Ruth Schlegel, and Debbie Kennedy, C.R.N.P., and Jane S. Zigenfus-Martin, C.N.M.

I deeply appreciate the birthing families who have given me moments of exquisite joy and nights of restless anguish, and I am grateful to the neighbors and community who have supported me.

Lastly I am thankful to Rich, who brought me home and keeps me safe.

PENELOPE BRADBURY ARMSTRONG, C.N.M.
LANCASTER COUNTY, PENNSYLVANIA
AUGUST 1985

I

Their Way

Here around Honeybrook it's hillier than where Richie and I live. Small woods are more common, the banks of the streams are higher, and the water runs with more snap. Fields rise quickly and disappear abruptly over low ridges. It's dark outside now, but soon the mist will start rising from the streams and will seep out to fill the hollows in the fields. The corn waits, stiff and crackling, for the farmers to get up and begin cutting. Most of the cows will still be settled on their knees before I leave this delivery, and at this time of year, it might even be eight o'clock before the ducks start dropping into the ponds.

Amos and Naomi's kitchen table, where I will fill out my paperwork, is covered with a green-and-white checked oilcloth, which has been scrubbed and left bare except for a glowing kerosene lantern. Amos is in the bedroom with Naomi, who's almost ready to have her baby. As soon as she's a little farther along, I'll go back into the bedroom and help her.

I've been delivering babies for Amish couples since

1979. I'm not Amish myself. In fact, I am, or was, about as "English," or non-Amish, as they come. That is to say, I was aggressive and willful. But I believe I'm becoming less so every day. I'm trying.

In the early months of my practice, I was enchanted with these people, the way I might become attached to a simple, engaging melody. It's easy for that to happen. Take this young Amishman, Amos; he's irresistible. For one thing, he is in splendid good health. Since he spends his days jumping on and off of his wagon; tossing around loads of hay or corn; pulling, carrying, lifting, and driving his team through his fields, he's strong and lithe. Then, too, I think he's a joy to watch, doing all his working and playing in black, baggy pants cut off short at the shins and held up by a pair of suspenders. Solid, bright-colored shirts make his shiny eyes seem even brighter than they actually are. His hair is cut bluntly just below the earlobes, and when he combs it, he parts it in the center and drags the comb dead flat against the curve of his head, as if to get the furrows straight. He wears a flat-brimmed, black felt hat for dress and a straw hat for fieldwork, and since he's married, he's got an untrimmed Abraham Lincoln beard.

The main thing, though, is his Amishman's face and eyes. "English" men, as the Amish call the rest of us, rarely have faces like these men. I think it's because the English always have to go to meetings where they must outmaneuver, outsmart, and beat the other fellows to the punch, whereas an Amishman's only meetings are on Sunday mornings in somebody's kitchen when he prays. An Amishman passes his day riding a wagon slung on leather straps, making agreements with the weather, and when he's done with that he has only to walk the path through the pole beans to get dinner with his family. In the silence of his farmhouse, before and after each meal, he drops his head, and prays silently.

An Amishman usually looks like something special is happening to him. He has the face of a boy who has been teaching ducks to swim in a metal tub and now he's come in to tell his mother about it, and while he talks, jumping around, she's taking cookies out of the oven.

Through an Amishman's eyes, the days look like handcrafted gifts from God—presents made of carved wood and string and parts that make a reedy whistle.

Consider Amos. I pulled into the lane tonight and had barely parked when the kitchen door opened and out he came, flashlight in hand, offering to help. I asked him to get the suitcase, so he picked up that forty-pound monstrosity the way I'd pick up a head of lettuce. Amos is a smart one. Calls me on the phone in the middle of the night and in his soft voice says, "Would you like to come to the grand opening of the Baby Outlet?" I imagine his eyes really shone when he said that.

Ha-ha, I thought.

The Amish like to write "ha-ha's" in their letters. I've grown fond of the ha-ha's myself.

It wasn't a bad line, especially for a farmer whose wife is in labor with their second baby and who had to walk down the lane and across a frost-crusted field to a phone shed to call the midwife. "Oh, it was just something I thought of saying as I was walking along," he says, delighted with himself.

Amos is a tease. Used to take his sister's dolls out behind the barn, put them in a shoe-box coffin, and bury them. "I only did it when somebody pulled a stump over on me," he says in idle defense.

"So you think you're going to get a baby out tonight?" I ask.

"Well, I wouldn't mind," he answers, showing me the way into the darkened house.

Amos and Naomi are typically Amish, except that just now they're living in what will be their stable. All this land around here was woodland until three or four years ago, when a bunch of older Amishmen got together and bought it—it's about the last tillable piece of land in the county—now they're selling it at low interest to young Amish couples who want to have their own farms.

Amos and Naomi settled here after they were married a few years ago and began to clear the land. Naomi, bandana on her head, black tennis shoes, bright-colored skirt clinging to her knees, black apron snapping in the wind, worked right alongside Amos —cutting, driving the team, hauling, and all the rest. I practically had to tie her to the stove to get her to lay off at the end of her first pregnancy. They felled the small forest that covered the land and collected the logs into a mountainous pile for selling, and then, with the help of their families, they began to work the land. Next summer they expect to get their house up.

An Amishman wants his farm more than anything. I've watched a man's eyes fill with tears when he talked about getting his own place. He wants to be with his family, to step over his children in the barn and work with them next to him in the field; he wants to have his father and mother in an attached house. He wants to be as intimate with his land as you and I might be with the palm of our hand.

4

* * *

Naomi put on a white batiste gown, lightly hand-quilted at the yoke. Her hair, parted severely down the center of her head and drawn into a knot at the back, was covered by a white kerchief. At least an hour before, Amos had crawled up on the bed next to her, and since then, his massive farmer's fingers dusted with baby powder, he'd been rubbing her back. Her whole body loosened up from the heat of labor and from his massaging.

I asked her to pull her knee directly up to her chin. She buried her fingers deep into the thigh of her leg and sank into a powerful push.

Since Naomi had so little extra weight on her, you could almost see the bones of her pelvis giving way to the force of her pushing. They spread slowly, grindingly and firmly, the way plates of the earth would move during a quake; they allowed the baby's head to pass downward, the shoulders to turn along the spiraling route to the outside world. Naomi waited, breathed deeply, took Amos's hand, and threw all her strength into her abdomen again, and as if burying a heavy rock there, she gave another push. I could see the top of the baby's head.

She pushed again and as the head crowned, the skin of the perineum stretched around it; the head moved closer to freedom and Naomi's skin thinned to transparency. I had worked the portal skin on the outside while the baby's head stretched it from the inside, and between the two of us we eased in all the stretch available. Naomi gave a series of short pushes, she panted, the baby's head shifted—and there was its forehead and the top of its brow and the face. The head made a quarter turn and Naomi—pausing only a moment—pushed out her new baby girl. I cut the cord, wrapped the baby quickly, and Amos grabbed it, cooing, chuckling, and hopping from side to side like a father bird. Later, when I took the baby out to the kitchen for a bath and I sudsed her head, I told her about how a long shaft of morning light was reaching across the kitchen countertop and making the faucet handles glow; how the windmill was creaking to life, pulling water from the well. I showed her, once I had the towel fluffed about her head, how the lawn, through the panes at the sink window, was iridescent, and I watched while the long branches of the protective yard oak stretched and lazily flapped. The morning was lavender and frost.

It takes a long time to learn the ways of another culture. When I first began practicing in Lancaster County, Pennsylvania, I suspected the Amish of being a cold, unfeeling people. I heard a story of a doctor who worked all night long in surgery to save the first-born infant son of an Amish couple. Shortly before dawn, the baby died and the doctor, wiping tears of exhaustion and defeat from his own eyes, told the couple their baby was gone.

Using very few words, they thanked him, said they believed they wouldn't be needed anymore at the hospital, and she put on her cape and bonnet and he put on his hat. Without crying, without calling out "Why?," without rending the hallways with their sorrow, they walked out.

A few weeks ago, I delivered my first stillborn child at home—my first death in a thousand births. Had it been five years ago, I would have been destroyed. I would have given up the work. I would not have known how to withstand the loss; I would have blamed myself; I would have known there was a way

I could have prevented it. In those days, I did not permit what I considered imperfection—either in myself or in the universe. I would have thrashed out, railed and stormed at the skies, if death had had the nerve to cross my path.

But I've been here too long, and even I—the most willfull of the willful—am slowly learning to be as courteous to death as I have always been toward birth. Not at all have I learned to be cold; rather, I've become more peaceful.

II 〰

Home

Maybe Grammy strode into my dream. Maybe one more time she grabbed me by the arm, dug her knuckles into my shoulder, and said, "Don't try any of those little-girl tricks with me, young lady. You want something done, you figure out how to do it yourself. You make something of yourself."

In any case, I woke up in the middle of the night with the answer. I sat up in bed for a long time, staring and wondering if it was as good as it seemed.

I walked downstairs, stoked up the fire in the wood stove, and paced back and forth in front of it.

"I think I'll be a midwife," I mumbled. "I'm going to be a midwife," I said aloud.

I knew it was right, although not by reasoning—I was a long way from being rational about my future. After all, I had already gone to college, I had a decent job, one that had earned me enough to make payments on my very own tiny farmhouse. On weekends and evenings over the past three years, I'd knocked down the old warped interior walls and nailed up used barn board; I'd brought in Vermont slate so the kitchen floor would look like the tide pools at Boothbay. I'd been to the dump and collected old bottles and set them on a dish rail. I'd bought my plates from my neighbor the potter and hung pots and pans from a rack made by my friend the blacksmith. I was at a point where I could serve a meal for friends.

Neither was my midwifery idea fashionable. I had my dream in 1974, and people didn't aspire to being midwives then. Widows in nineteenth-century novels did, a few leftover hippies maybe. People would think I'd been reading an unexpurgated version of the *Whole Earth Catalogue*.

But I'd met somebody recently who was a midwife and I'd been thinking about the idea. And besides, when I was in high school, I would wait until after everyone went to bed and then I'd crawl out the window, sneak out to the car, let it roll down the driveway, start it up, and drive to the emergency ward of the local hospital so I could watch medical dramas. That must have meant something.

"Of course," I said to myself, "'The Squire of Brentwood' proves it." That was a paper I wrote in high school. We had sheep at home then (the Squire was a most prolific ram), and I wrote a paper in my English class about how I couldn't concentrate on writing a paper because I'd been up all night with my arm inside a sheep's uterus. "All activities pale"— I remembered writing something grandiose like that—"when compared to the excitement of the maternity ward."

The heart of it was, though, that being a midwife went along with everything I believed in. If I became a midwife, I could help give other families a start toward being like mine had been.

In other words, it came out of Nana's kitchen.

Nana's kitchen was the way things were supposed to be. It had Nana's lap. It also had a rocking chair, a Seth Thomas clock, and it hummed with the lives of women who bustled, scrubbed, patted, mended, and arranged. Women whose entire lives were concerned with their homes, husbands, children, family, friends, and neighbors.

Nana and Pappy had started with nothing but their youth and Yankee values. In the winters, Pappy worked in the Maine woods, sleeping with eleven men on one long straw mattress, and in summers he hired out on farms until he had enough money to buy the land on Westford Hill, Hodgdon Corners, Aroostook County, Maine. The original white frame farmhouse, with its kitchen, parlor, and two upstairs bedrooms, went up in 1912. My mom was born there; so were her brother and sister. I was there the night my brother was born in 1948.

In Nana's kitchen I learned about woman's work. Nana taught me to garden, cook, bake, and preserve. On long summer afternoons, with aunts, she-cousins, and neighbors all moving softly about, bumping plump, pasty arms, I learned the rich satisfaction of tiering pears and peaches in mason jars; I came to savor the sweet steam rising from the pots; and wandering away from the edges of industry, I developed an affection for the piles of pits and peelings whose colors grew deeper and darker throughout the sweltering afternoons.

The women were sinking values into my bones. Not with their words, but with the smell of bubbling butter, brown sugar, and cinnamon; the rhythm of fingers turning and flying across a pie crust; the sound of their voices moving in and out of the sound of their work; the room underfoot and on step stools they made for me. I became like them, before words, before thought.

Nana formed me with abundant and unconditional love. At the kitchen table, she'd show me how to cut out and sew pajamas with one snap in the front for my dolls, and while we worked she'd say over and over again, "You can get yourself into any trouble whatsoever, young lady, go ahead and try. It won't make any difference. I'll love you and you can't help yourself."

Fortunately for my patients today, my mother's ideas about responsibility more than balanced Nana's breakaway heart. Mother was interested in standards —stern ones, ones that did not give way to stories, excuses, or extenuating circumstances. When I did something wrong, she sent me directly to my room, where I could concentrate, undisturbed and uncomforted, about my misdeed. Gradually I understood that responsibility is absolute and personal; that there's no shrugging it off when things become difficult.

If there had just been Nana, I would probably be a plump, contented farm wife today. But I had Grammy. Grammy was my great-grandmother on my dad's side. Grammy, the woman who raised my father, had no interest in punch and cookies.

Grammy smoked a pipe, spit, wore rouge and bangled earrings, and sang dirty ditties. She ranted and raged at the whole pissant, goddam mean world. She was massive. Her breasts were so big and so undisciplined that she had to hold them up with one forearm in order to get her belt buckled underneath. I thought she was spectacular.

We have one old brown photo of Grammy as a

young woman. There's a log cabin sitting no-non-sense in the middle of the picture. Grammy's young family is lined up in front of it. Miserable, cold-looking leaves are straying all over the ground. Another bleak November in the Maine woods; nothing to look forward to but five months of life-threatening cold.

Grammy's husband is over to the right. Although he must have been a fairly young man, his shoulders had already eroded. He had his pants hitched up and cinched. He didn't exactly glare at the photographer, but it's no smile either. Posing for the picture was clearly only one more miserable activity in his scabby, itchy, cold, dirty, and mean lifetime. Must be his 30-30 leaned up against the wall of the cabin.

A step or two away from him is Grammy. An Amazon. Her hair is drawn up high in a knot; her dress is a fortress, seamed with rivets from shoulder to ground. For the purposes of the picture, she'd set the butt of her gun firmly on the ground and rested her hand ever so comfortably on its barrel.

One of the little girls standing near Grammy would be my father's mother—but it wasn't she who raised my father. For involved reasons, Grammy did that.

I loved Grammy. I was absolutely fascinated by her. Grammy—crude, tough, and vulgar—was a midwife.

III ❧

Midwife

"*Nurse Bradburry*," she would say in her stiff brogue. "Recite for me the mechanisms for a left occipito-anterior presentation."

I would rise, step into the aisle to the left of my desk, smooth the hard white canvas of my nurse's skirt, fold my hands in front of me, look directly ahead, and respond to the instructor.

"Thank you, Miss Helms. The mechanisms for the left occipito-anterior delivery are..." And so it went—right occipito-anterior, frank breech, footling breech, left occipito-posterior. We recited, repeated, and tapped the words into our skulls as if by mallet and awl.

By the time I could roll out the answers like that, I'd been at Highlands General Hospital in Scotland for almost eight months. I'd completed my preparation for midwifery training: a one-year intensive course in nursing in Saint Louis, Missouri, followed by six months of probationary nursing at Highlands. Of course, the six months had seemed more like an advanced form of hazing than a probation. When I first got to Scotland and the cabbie let me off at the dark medieval door of the hospital, he rolled his eyes and looked at me as if I were condemned.

A "matron" greeted me. "Block thirty-seven," she said, jangling her keys. "Follow me." She led me to a cell fitted with a sink, four hangers, and a beige clay jar, meant for warming my feet. I looked at the iron bedstead, undoubtedly left over from the early days of the maternity hospital at Highlands. I'd read about those beds.

> Throughout history most babies were born at home. Maternity hospitals were first started for homeless women and were really extensions of poorhouses... These first maternity hospitals were convenient centers for medical students to learn and practice obstetrics, but infections were rampant, as doctors conveyed bacteria on their hands from one patient to another, and many babies and mothers died. They were possibly the most dangerous places in which women could possibly give birth.*

I crawled into the bed every night, bidding sweet dreams to all the women who had died of septicemia in it, and then, in the mornings, I would apply myself to perfecting my use of the sterile trolley. As far as I could tell, the sterile trolley was the one overriding ritual of nursing in the United Kingdom.

One did not nurse without the sterile trolley. Suppose for example, one wished to apply a Band-Aid to a patient's wound. One would pull out the trolley and fall upon it with a scrub brush and a noxious-smell-

*Sheila Kitzinger, *The Complete Book of Pregnancy and Childbirth* (New York: Alfred A. Knopf, 1983), p. 38.

ing foam. Once one had scrubbed the trolley, one draped it. Once one draped it, one could set out one's bowl. Then one could set out another and another. The bowls were followed by scissors, gauze, syringes, needles, clamps, calculator, butterfly nets, tubs of margarine, and I cannot remember what else, except for the Band-Aid. Once this procedure had been observed, one could apply the Band-Aid. Needless to say, if one touched anything while one was setting up one's trolley, if one broke the sterile field, one started over again—"straightaway."

Each day I took my maidenly trolley into the male urology ward, where the sun didn't shine. I must elaborate. The sun didn't shine for five months. It was a filthy, smelly, and dingy place. Every few days, they dragged a cold mop down the center aisle, leaving wax curled up like old men's toenails in the corners of the rooms and under the beds. They never washed the windows, as far as I could tell, and there were no screens, so when the days grew warmer, the flies came in and settled on the patients' wounds.

The men lay in bed after bed—ten down one side, nine back up the other. Nineteen iron beds and nineteen iron grates. I gave nineteen sick men—victims of strokes, men with cancer crawling from the inside out—baths every day. There wasn't one shower for the entire ward. They each peed for me in glass urinals, which I placed in a wooden cart and pulled, rattling, behind me. Then I tested the nineteen samples and scrubbed the urinals clean.

I learned a new nursing vocabulary, one made up of singularly revolting words. For example, an IV was no longer called an IV; it was to be called a "drip." Gastric suction was called—I do not invent—a "suck." Which made the treatment for gastric distress a "drip and suck."

The rain and wind blew directly down off the Highlands and rattled the window of my room each day for that entire time. The other students ignored me, and my energy, generously inspired though it was, dwindled. Fortunately, in June, five months after my arrival, they announced that I would be granted my license as a nurse in the United Kingdom, and that after a summer holiday in America, I could begin midwifery training. I'd made it to the good part.

By the time I returned to Glasgow in the fall, I had read and reread Maggie Myles's *Textbook for Midwives* so many times that I knew her words backward and forward and I ached to talk about what I'd learned, to challenge and question. I found, to my great frustration, that there was to be none of it. Not only did the system discourage inquiry, the students themselves seemed to resent it. When I'd mention something about what we'd learned to one of my classmates, I'd be dismissed with a look of annoyance. Finally, I realized that the typical student at Highlands was there because it gave her a chance for a promotion at home, or maybe a chance to get to America; she was unlikely to have much interest in midwifery itself. It was best to go about one's work dull-eyed and perfunctory.

Since I couldn't find someone with whom to share my enthusiasm, I retreated into myself. I ran every day, and on holidays I rode the bus to the Highlands, and while reviewing the positions a baby could take in the birth canal—left occipito, right occipito—I walked endless miles through heather. I pictured every turn, every bump on the road in the birth passage. I imagined changes in pressure and the way they would feel to the baby's head and shoulders passing by. I imagined the mother's muscles weaving supple, powerful slings to help her child out. I would come back to the library from my walks and search for answers to questions I'd discovered while making imaginary deliveries.

I went to class and recited my lessons. I tried to eat well. I hung around the delivery room. I read Maggie Myles again. Like the woman whose baby I would deliver, I roamed restlessly in the last weeks before my first baby.

Finally, they called me to meet the woman. Her long, angular face reached at least a half a head higher than her husband's. She had a bristly thatch of hair on her chin, uneven brows, big bones, and dark blotches on her skin. Her eyes bulged slightly, and later, when she pulled in her breath during contractions, her cheeks sank into graceful hollows, as if they'd been carved by a slow-running waterfall. Her legs were ribbed with strength. I thought Janet was very beautiful.

She'd put on a freshly starched and ironed smock to wear to the hospital, and since she was very nervous, she held tightly to her husband's arm. He stayed with her throughout. "It's our first, you know," he said, patting her hand. In his shirt pocket were two three-by-five cards: the first one had the choices of the baby's names; on the second, Janet had written the names and phone numbers of all the relatives he was to call. He pulled the cards out and showed them to me.

As her labor progressed and the contractions increased, she began to whistle through them; she'd be talking, then she'd slow down, roll up and over and perch on her right elbow, suck in her breath, and whistle a few bars of a tune I couldn't make out. She was a determined girl. I don't think she had the faintest idea she was whistling.

Her husband let her pull on him, tug at him, and dig her fingernails into his palm. Once or twice toward the end she said she couldn't go on, that it couldn't be done, but he'd stroke her hair and tell her softly, "Don't look now, gal, but you are already doing it."

When she got to the point where she wanted to push, we moved her to the delivery room, and before long she was at the last of it.

I watched the top of the head coming toward me in laps, moving forward during a contraction, then dropping back. I had studied it so much, I could feel the mechanism of the birth canal—the rhythm of turning, burrowing, climbing, clenching, and easing—as the baby secured his path. I longed to put my hand on Janet's belly to assure myself that the way I knew it felt was the way it felt.

She gripped the sides of her cot. I massaged the perineum. The head crowned. I touched the tips of my fingers to the creamy scalp and felt the pulse. Time stopped and I stopped and my hands joined with the baby's head. The baby's face crept out from under its mother's covering of skin. As the head came, my fingers eased along the cheeks almost as if a groove had been worn there to guide me. My fingers slid beneath the chin. The world turned then, one time and one time only on the axis made by the baby's head and body. Then the baby floated out into my hands.

Janet whistled ever so lightly, and beneath my mask I smiled, because from the moment I touched the child's head I knew I had been born to be a midwife.

IV ❧

Wifie

Even though I hated the place, I learned a lot at Highlands General Hospital. I delivered babies. I thought nothing of working a seven-to-four shift, then sleeping and eating and coming back for an eleven-to-eight. I talked them into giving me extra time in labor and less time in the nursery. I lived my life at the doors of the delivery room hoping they would need an extra pair of hands. Happily I was part stewardess, part nurse, and part general delivery mechanic. Contentedly I scrubbed up, set up, and tore down. Eagerly I delivered big babies, little babies, flat babies, eager babies, preemies, twins. I did three breech deliveries in my first twenty. By the time I left Glasgow, I'd caught forty babies.

I learned one skill poorly taught in the United States—how to use my hands to best advantage—but I worked under a medical style that I vowed to combat wherever I encountered it.

At Highlands Hospital, form ranked above everything else, including the well-being of the mother and child. Form, indifferent as it might be to need, was the thing. I should have figured it out from the sterile trolley business.

In the first place, a woman was to have her baby on time. Not when her body indicated, not when the baby had matured, but when the calendar prescribed. If a woman hadn't delivered by her due date, "Pop you go into the hospital, girl, and we'll get this wee motor revved up now, won't we?"

The machinery started. It was incredible. There's not enough money in all of Scotland to bring in a bunch of fresh broccoli, but every last obstetric gadget in the modern world is automatically hooked up to a woman having a baby. First they put a catheter to her bladder. Then they put two wiry probes into her vagina: one is placed in the uterus to measure contractions, and the other is screwed into the baby's scalp to measure the fetal heartbeat. Contractions and beats follow the wire out to a metal box, which translates them onto a continuous band of paper. When the doctors come in to check a woman, they do not look at her, ask her questions, or feel her belly; they read the graph paper coming out of her machine.

Finally, she is given an IV with Pitocin, a drug that causes contractions to start or grow stronger, and once it's going, she has until the end of the shift to get into action. If she hasn't had her baby by then, they give her an anesthetic and boost up the Pitocin —a combination which, incidentally, slows down the baby's heartbeat. In the second shift, she is to be ready to push. If she isn't, she's posted for cesarean section.

If she is ready to push, however—if her body should choose to be in harmony with the schedule of

Highlands General Hospital—she goes to the delivery room. She doesn't actually go; she rides lickety-split on a metal trolley, crashing into walls and doorways on the way—a kind of permanent hysteria rules the corridors—and then she is lifted from the trolley to the delivery table, to which she is secured by tethers and ties. Her private parts are scrubbed. Her unscrubbed parts are covered with sterile draping.

The midwives scrub too: hot water, a soft brush, and iodine for fifteen minutes. We hold our hands up the entire time to keep the soiled water from dripping back onto them. Assistants help us with gowns and we dive our hands upward into sterile gloves. Then we set up the sterile trolley: forty instruments in order. And if we fail to do that just so, then, yes, everything comes apart again, never mind the woman having a baby.

No one asks what one is to do if it is a choice between the sterile trolley and the life of the baby. The idea is not to deliver babies, but to become a perfect mechanism in the delivery room.

Sister directs everything. We do as we are told. We do things we have never heard of; we do things we know are harmful. I had one baby whose face showed deep blue and whose neck was bound by three tight loops of the umbilical cord: a baby in severe distress. I slipped clamps under the cord to cut it—a proper procedure, but, as Sister took pains to point out, done from the "wrong" side.

Never mind the oxygen loss to the baby. Never mind potential brain damage. Sister insisted that I remove the clamps and put them under the cord from the "right" side. So I did.

I watched while another student midwife tried to free a baby whose shoulder had stuck behind his mother's pubic bone. Like the baby whose neck is noosed by the cord, this baby was also suffering from oxygen deprivation. He needed the help of extraordinarily deft, strong, and experienced hands, but Sister was not scrubbed so Sister did not intervene. She gave instructions from the doorway while the student midwife groped and the baby suffered damage.

Most of the babies, having been drugged through their mother's bloodstream, were sluggish at birth and we had to blow up their lungs for them before they were willing to breathe. I thought all babies were born like that, resisting birth, having to be convinced to live. Subconsciously, it must have made some sense to me. Who would want to be born in Glasgow?

By and large, the women came from hideous lives. Some of them knew instinctively that their children's lives would be too brutal to be justifiable. So, in ways that were eruptive, gross, and thick—the only way they knew—they resisted reproduction. "Poor wifies" we called them, poor women of Glasgow who would reach down with their hands and try to force their baby's head back into the womb when they could feel it being born.

Some fought with all their strength.

Margaret, a thin, rodent-faced creature, came to us filled with loathing. Her sister and mother pulled her through the door, explaining and reexplaining to anyone who showed even vague interest: "She says she don't want no baby; she always said she never did want no baby. Said she never did have anything for herself when she was growing up and she was going to have something when she was grown. All she ever talked about was saving her money so she could move to London and live decent. I'd say she thought she was a little better than the rest of us, but I guess she found out she was just the same."

I was kind to her, thinking I might give her a small measure of the respect she so desperately sought. She screamed back at me how she didn't need any consideration from people like me. She'd taken care of herself just fine without my help up to now and nothing would please her more than if I'd just go hang.

As the labor progressed, her raving and kicking grew more violent. She'd hiss and spit and beat us away when we tried to go near her to examine her.

"I won't have this baby. I won't have it. Never. No one can make me." And she'd swing out at anyone who dared close in on her bed.

I saw her baby's head crowning and thought she'd be enough distracted by the pain so that I could dart in to catch it, but in a moving show of will, she jumped from her bed and ran down the hall. I followed, pace for pace, my hands help up for sterility. Nurses in the hall backed up flat against the walls in shock.

I chased her a half a block down the dimly lit hallway, the baby turning out as we ran; I chased her until she reached a dead end. She turned toward me, preparing, I could tell from the snarl on her lip, to fight dirty. I thought, How could I get the baby out without hurting it or her? I turned around too, and backing up against her, pinning her to the wall, I reached through my own legs and hers and—as if in a reverse football "hike"—I took her baby from her. We walked back to the room, both of us silent, the baby in my arms, the cord between us, the placenta still in her.

* * *

For six weeks of our training, we did "district" postpartum care. We checked in each morning at the hospital, and wrapped in massive blue cloaks, high-black shoes, and starched white hats, we took our list of addresses for that day's follow-up visits.

We wandered through all the back streets and burnt-out tenements of Glasgow.

We carried rolls of newspapers to spread out in the flats we visited, to protect ourselves, our babies, and whatever open wounds we found. We wore huge rubber aprons. That way, when we went to homes where there were no basins in which to wash the babies, we could fill our laps with warm water and bathe the babies in them.

I'd reach the base of some dark suitcase, putrid with filth, and call out the name of the woman I was seeking. Generally, a man's voice would hurtle back like a rusty missile, "Who's there?"

"Nurse Bradbury," I'd respond.

His voice would change. Our position gave us protection. (We were highly respected. We seldom paid for coffee at the counter or for bus fare. Drunks would raise on an elbow to salute us as we passed. We appeared to be bold, but we were safe in the jungle.) "Come up, Sister," he would say.

Unfortunately, what I had to say and teach my new mothers was not similarly respected. Teaching was impossible. Poverty, ignorance, and brutality preceded me and my lessons. What I taught dissolved instantly in the foul inheritance. Standing at a greasy sink, a baby in my arms, looking for a spot—any spot—to put down newspapers, a timid wifie crouched at my elbow and a vile man saying, "She doesn't need to know how to wash the bairn'," I vanished into a memory of Nana's kitchen, with its white starched and ruffled curtains, its Seth Thomas clock ticking, its rocking chair. Nana's kitchen lived inside me, gave me comfort, and guided me toward the way things should be.

Then I looked at the man standing there, his pants half zipped, his bare white hairy arm leaning on the countertop, his eyes puffy and red, and tried to remember that his mother probably knew to try to push him back in.

We counseled women on family planning; we fit them for a diaphragm and carefully explained how important it was to use it every time they had intercourse. A month or two later they'd be in the clinic, pregnant.

"What happened?"

"It was my neighbor's turn to use the diaphragm," she'd say, "and my husband, he didn't want to wait."

Men, using kitchen knives and claiming their "rights," would cut open their wives' stitches.

I was as kind and gentle as I could be while I was with the women. I talked to them about how to keep the baby warm and its tummy full. I answered their questions as best I could. That was all I could do. The system was fixed; everybody had to stay and do and be what they were, and had been now and forever, in the hospital and out.

V

Booth

In Philadelphia, driving down City Line Drive from the north, you'll notice a change from ordinary city to blue-blood suburbs. Notice Saint Joseph's College* on your left, its entry fronted by a well-kept half circle of lawn, trimmed with flowers. On the right, down a long, broad sidewalk shaded by elms, is the Jesuit sanctuary. A stone-and-iron fence lines the sidewalk and the grass rolls comfortably back into havens of silence, meditation, and profound thought. Further along are domesticated glens, ravines, and meadows where sunlight puddles and splashes.

America. Soft, bountiful, sunny, generous, democratic, land-of-fresh-vegetables America.

I was coming home. I had certification as a nurse-midwife in the United Kingdom. I had yet to be licensed for practice in the United States; that would take sixteen weeks of training at Booth Maternity Center on City Line Drive in Philadelphia.

*The names in this chapter have not been changed nor have any of the events been altered.

Booth began as a home for unwed mothers with a maternity hospital attached. Birth control pills, safe abortions, and tolerance for single parents forced Booth either to change its services or go out of business. A physician, John Franklin, proposed a plan for family-centered maternity care.

His idea, considered radical in 1971, when he offered it, was that childbirth was a normal event for the body and a normal, important event for the family. Believing that medical technology was used too commonly and casually in childbirth, he argued that it disrupted the harmony between the mother and her body, her baby's birth and her family. "We wanted to support the mother's own heartfelt instincts for her baby and to see if we can graft on care as good as the maximum intervention kind of delivery service." He proposed a hospital delivery style, using a nurse-midwife/physician team, which he thought would be healthier for the mother, the child, and the family. The local Maternity Center Association, the Salvation Army, and the people at Booth joined with Franklin and created one of the most innovative and caring maternity hospitals in the nation.

I flew home at spring break at Highlands and interviewed with Sue Yates, Booth's Director of Education. I approached the crumbling old Main Line mansion. At the entry, there is a circular drive with a weedy bed in the center. A dogwood tree thrives there now, nourished by placentas planted by students of a graduating class after mine. Two or three steps lead up to the Queen Anne porch. The hand-plastered walls are the color of egg cream; and the tiles, where they haven't slipped away, are red. In winter, there's just the massive oak door facing you. In summertime, a wide, swaying screen door would be banging open and shut.

I went into a parlor. The mantelpiece was buffed; the fireplace appeared to work; and gray couches were filled with fluffy pillows. Sun streamed from the adjoining rooms, where Sue Yates had her office.

"The Booth experience," Sue Yates said, "is very demanding. You have to have your eyes open and be ready to go. You can't be depressed, or upset, or distracted by any other major responsibilities." She wanted to know if I could arrange my life around such a program.

From where I sat, I could see a wall full of books, periodicals, and texts. I knew that in the next room there were shelves filled with more books, periodicals, tapes, plastic models of women's bellies with doll babies to go in and out of them, and videotaped lectures on all aspects of childbirth from experts around the world. This included my old friend Maggie Myles making her world-famous "Hands Off the Breech" speech.

My mouth watered. Could I arrange my life? Could I arrange my life to be in a place where they wanted me to learn everything that I could about delivering babies? Sue Yates had no idea how easily I could do that.

"It is not only the schedule," she said. "There is—no matter what one's training—professional culture shock. If your experience has been in a high-tech hospital, then our laid-back ways make you question our performance standards; if your experience has been laid back, then our precision is irritating."

The student midwives at Booth come from all over the world, most of them to get their certification in

America. Each one, she explained, has certain personal and cultural limits to overcome. One Irish woman, "a lovely, elegant, long-necked girl," was extremely competent in the delivery room, Sue said, but she balked and crumbled when children attended a birth. The prospect of giving sex counseling or discussing veneral disease gave her a sick headache.

"A Chilean woman," she continued, "who had practiced independently for many years had a deep interest in therapeutic touch and holistic healing. She was initially offended by our use of technology, which she thought barbaric."

"Finally," she said, "we demand self-reliance and self-criticism of our students. We find that nurses are accustomed to deferring to physicians, so they have difficulty in assuming complete responsibility for the outcome of their work, let alone the responsibility of advocating for patients in the face of an unsympathetic medical community. This business of being independent and professionally responsible is even more difficult for midwives coming out of more hierarchical settings—like those in the United Kingdom, for example."

Amen, I said to myself, thinking of Sister standing at the door of the delivery room with her hands clasped politely in front of her while the baby degenerated.

I felt wonderfully, blissfully at home. I told her calmly and convincingly that I was strenuously self-reliant. I told her I wanted the premium training that Booth was reputed to give. I told her I had made considerable sacrifices to go this far, that I had a demonstrated record of singleness of purpose, and that I intended to be excellent. Booth could help me be excellent. I told her I needed the certification.

I didn't tell her that the most attractive man I'd ever met had just taken a job flying for a commuter airline out of Philly.

She said I could come, and so, six days after I returned to the United States from Glasgow, I began my course at Booth.

Booth *was* demanding. It *was* a culture shock. As given as I was to being independent, to running my own show, to making my own decisions, to an emergency room mentality, I found it wrenching to transform myself immediately from delivery room wind-up nurse to professional midwife. I even wondered in that first week or so if I shouldn't have waited for the next class. But the feeling didn't last. Instead of taking strength out of me, Booth nourished me, gave me confidence, and rewarded my skill. The people there wanted me to learn and to take good care of mothers —the very things I was most determined to do well.

First of all, they let us learn everywhere and under any circumstances. Not only in the library in the house, but in the hospital, too. There were funky cubbyholes, closets really, with coffee and ashtrays, tables and chairs where we could sit, talk, sketch anatomies and maneuvers on the tabletop, and fight about how such and such a delivery should have been done. We debated the degree of technical intervention that was best. Do you drug them or not? What do you do, for example, with a Byrn Mawr type who isn't willing to give herself up to you; women who, instead of saying, "Oh, Penny, you can get me through this?" would say, "You have no right to push me through this." We were constantly plotting and analyzing the way different women would have their babies.

Everything was different here. It was human.

Everybody—mothers, babies, siblings, midwives, doctors—all of us were supposed to be regular people with lives around us. Our families, our hobbies, our busted radiators, impossible mothers-in-law, floated in and out of our work. Our human side was allowed to show: take Sue Yates giving an introductory slide show about siblings at a birth. She was the consummate professional; she was in charge, in control, and I expected her to behave that way—formal, highly disciplined, and always to the point.

What happens? She's giving her lecture, when up comes a slide of a kid who'd just watched his sister being born. Does she say, "We've included this slide so that you can see that children who attend births can feel comfortable and relaxed about the experience"? No. Instead her voice starts zooming along like a roller coaster on a downhill turn.

"Look at the kid," she says, as if she'd never seen the likes of him before. "Would you look at that kid?" She walks up a little closer to the screen and looks herself. The kid, a sibling of the newborn, is looking cute, that for sure. He's sitting in an oversized green hospital smock, in an oversized chair, with a brand new baby comfortably in his lap and with his scruffy old mud-puddle tennis shoes sticking out at the bottom of the smock. "Look at those feet!" she says, like it was her first grandson or something. She just liked the kid; that was her "professional" point.

The people at Booth had thorough respect and affection for women, for their families, and for their way of life. The women came from every imaginable local culture: Philadelphia Main Line, Black Muslims with their robes and beads and bongos, revolutionaries, blacks, Chicanos, Puerto Ricans, macrobiotic types, hippies, and preppies.

The prenatal clinic was a showroom for the maternity art done by the mothers: sketches, photographs, and watercolor washes portrayed women in labor, in delivery, and taking care of their families. Sculptures lined the windowsills—some wooden and primitive, totemic in quality; others troubled. I remember a small, bound-up female figure, for example, made of twisted and layered wire with a twisted-and-layered-wire fetus inside of her. A square wooden pregnant woman, not much different in liveliness than the square wooden chair she was glued to, was painted shiny, like a disco dancing boot, in white acrylic.

Birthing style was mother's choice. You could have your contractions in a standard hospital bed where the mattress would go into modifications of the rickrack position by the mere pushing of a button, in a room where there were fetal monitors, belly bands, epidurals, spinals, and locals. When you were ready to deliver, you could ride from there to the delivery room with its oxygen, stainless-steel rolling carts, plastic hoses, readouts, clamps, sutures, and shiny lights. Or you could have your baby in the birthing room, in an ordinary old Salvation Army bed with flowered sheets, friends massaging your back, and with your toddler sitting cross-legged beside you.

We meant for the woman's birthgiving to strengthen the identity and unity of her family and her way of life. So, for example, Southeast Asian families were welcome to move into the hospital with the patient. They lived on mats on the floor and cooked the mother's food. I remember especially a Korean woman whose family stewed up her afterbirth so she could drink the broth and, according to her belief, return the strength to her body that was lost in childbirth.

Although we couldn't accommodate crowds, we tried to fit in whomever the woman wanted at her birth. One woman wanted her boyfriend to bring his entire reggae band. Since there wasn't enough room indoors, the band played outside on the patio and the drummer stayed inside with us and beat his rhythms on the fetal monitor.

As in Glasgow, we delivered the babies of angry, hurt women. Viciously angry women. Women who probably had been having sexual relations since they were ten, but who had not had a vaginal examination until they arrived at our doorstep. I would explain about how I was going to examine them and then as gently as I possibly could, I would reach my fingers into their vagina.

They would scream, "Rape, rape, she's trying to rape me," and then kick and hit. For some of them, the fury persisted through prenatal care and all the way through delivery. They would hurl obscenities at the babies' fathers. "That son of a bitch did this to me. I'll kill him. I hate his baby. Take this fuckin' baby out of me and get rid of it." And once again, as with the wifies, there was a solid logic in their fury.

We had women who tried to make it work with their partners and brought them to the delivery, only to have them pass out from an overdose on the delivery room floor.

It wasn't much of a compensation, but we did work especially hard with those young inner-city mothers, girls of fourteen and fifteen who would let us help them. Booth's philosophy was to try to give them a good birth experience; to give them perhaps an altered view of what having a family might be like; let them see that it might not all be brutal. We stayed close to these girls, we avoided doping them up and wiring them up, not because they were less entitled to intervention, but because they were less informed consumers.

It is a well-educated middle-class woman came in to have natural childbirth and she decided halfway through to throw in the rag, that was her business. She'd read the baby manuals; she knew that some of the drugs would be passed on to her baby. But an inner-city fourteen-year-old couldn't really give an informed consent. She'd never taken Physiology 101 and didn't know that drugs traveled through her to her baby. She didn't know that she might be losing the first moments of touching her baby and having him or her look back at her with bright eyes. We coached the young girls, put cool cloths on their brows, brought them juice, and massaged their backs. We got to know them. Those of us who were able to, cooed to them. We helped them respect their body and its way of doing things.

I couldn't have given you any hard evidence, but it seemed that their births went better.

What was true before birth—the most homelike atmosphere possible—followed afterward. The postpartum floor—in most hospitals, a quiet, "hush, the babies are sleeping" twilight place—was jovial and hearty. Women would be padding up and down the halls or sitting in rocking chairs in their rooms with their babies; men would be wandering about at all hours, helping out, looking for things, smiling stupidly into space, taking their newborns for a walk down the corridors. The nursery, instead of being draped and closed up except for hospital regulation viewing hours, had no curtains. Typically a soft, shapeless, white-haired old woman in a calico apron would be there puttering around and talking to the new mothers, showing them how to bathe their new babies. The prints on the walls were taken from old children's storybooks from around the world: "Then hush a bye, sweet to the spell and song of the dream shell."

In the after-care program, the same attitude prevailed. The women—single, married, rich, poor, battered, loved, in babushkas or feathered hair dressings, ignorant of being a parent or overread and overeducated—were treated (with their babies, their partners, and their other children) as an honorable institution. They were a family, and that, at Booth, was the important thing.

If the women were respected, if their bodies were respected, so were we. Midwives at Booth delivered the babies. We needed the doctors there; we wanted the doctors there for complications and medical problems; but we handled the normal births. They would put their head in the delivery room door and ask if everything was okay; would they be needed?

We learned responsibility, some of us with difficulty, others easily. We did learn to be self-reliant. We were our patients' advocates. We had to assume professional responsibility for their well-being, even if it meant challenging the physicians. And we would have to do that. All of us. They didn't let us forget it. The American doctor, they taught us, was not keen on our opinions or our ways of delivering babies.

VI ❧

Paradise Visited

It would have been all right to have stayed at Booth as a resident midwife. Not only did I like Booth, but I had Richie nearby; he even went to Midwifery Association meetings with me. He was settled in a comfortable room in a big old boardinghouse, and pretty much thrilled at the idea that he was driving people around in the sky. While Richie flew, I got to do a lot of deliveries in a humane hospital.

The trouble was, Booth had taught me to question what I was doing. For example, in our cubbyhole discussions at Booth, other midwives would sometimes argue from a book called *Spiritual Midwifery*. "They say don't rupture the membranes until . . ." or "They say there is no such thing as an arrested labor." I learned that *Spiritual Midwifery* was a book written by a hippie midwife for a colony of hippies who'd followed "Stephen" in a bus from Berkeley and settled on farms in Tennessee. I knew they intervened in deliveries far less than we did and they depended a lot on the relationship of the midwife to the mother. In hippie talk, that was a "birthing energy" issue.

I'd consciously avoided buying the book. I suspected the author understood some processes better than we did in the hospital, but they were things I didn't want to have to work out while I was studying at Booth. Also, I had a good idea that "spiritual midwives" might be flaky; I'd seen so many flat babies— that is, babies who were slow to breathe—so many mothers whose labors had just plain stopped, to believe that you could safely and sensibly deliver babies on somebody's porch.

But I kept thinking about how *Spiritual Midwifery* said that a woman did better if her birth people stayed with her all the way through: "The Vow of the Midwife has to be that she will put out one hundred percent of her energy to the mother and the child that she is delivering until she is certain that they have safely made the passage."*

I didn't care for the hippie vow, but I was having a terrible time leaving women before they had their babies. I'd just get to the point where the woman's body and mind were intertwined with mine and she was trusting me and we were beginning to work together like we'd been at it for a lifetime, and I'd look at my watch. "End of my shift, girl," I was supposed to say in Glasgow style and then walk off. Every time I had to do it, I felt as if I'd wronged the mother and her child.

*Ina May Gaskin, *Spiritual Midwifery* rev. ed. (Summertown, Tenn.: The Book Publishing Company, 1980), p. 283. Gaskin and other midwives on "the Farm" are lay midwives; that is, their training is empirical or based on firsthand experience. The certified nurse-midwife, or C.N.M., on the other hand, must complete an approved course of study in both nursing and midwifery and be licensed to practice in her state.

* * *

I was leaning on the counter at the nurses' station, staring blankly into space, when the phone rang, a nurse talked for a minute, then put her hand over the mouthpiece. "Some G.P. out in the boonies wants to know if we have any midwives who want to come join him in his private practice, including home deliveries. Anybody here want to talk to him?"

"Why not?" I said.

I had never been to Pennsylvania Dutch country. Amish, Mennonites, Hutterites, plain people, farmers, cultists, whatever—it was all the same to me. I had seen pictures in *National Geographic* of women wearing below-the-knee dresses and aprons; of men with beards who farmed with horses. Everybody was supposed to drive around in buggies instead of cars. One image stood out—a line of buggies in procession across a hill at sunset. I thought the whole thing was a little overdone, but what could I say? At Booth I'd learned some tolerance.

I drove out the Pennsylvania Turnpike on a cloudless morning. I was contented, looking forward to a break in routine. I buzzed along, cutting in and out of traffic. An hour later, at exit 23, I pulled off the turnpike. A matching pair of two-story brick houses with Federalist porticoes and green shutters faced me across the intersection. In this part of Pennsylvania— that is, anywhere within a fifty-mile radius of Gettysburg—you feel like you're about to see either an eighteenth-century cannonball hurtling over a stone wall or George Washington himself. What I saw, actually, besides the Revolutionary homes, were gas station signs and restaurant billboards.

I was on my way to Intercourse. Dr. Kaufman's

office was in Paradise, but I figured that as long as I was coming out this way, I would go to Intercourse, which is a village in the heart of Amish country. It's impossible not to be curious about a place named Intercourse.

On second glance, the restaurant billboards didn't look the same anymore; they were simpler and cruder than they would be in Gettysburg. That was serious indication that I was getting near the country. I drove past a row of trees, a few more brick homes, a vacant lot—and then farmhouses started appearing by the side of the road.

These weren't just any old farmhouses, they were white two-story farmhouses like in the old Maine—farmhouses with barbered lawns and immaculate flower beds. Grape vines, not yet showing any leaves, were pinned in swags to porch roofs and were waiting there patiently for warmer days. Neat concrete paths led in a straight line to each front door and even here, along a major thoroughfare, the dirt between the edge of the roads and the edge of the lawns was marked by the teeth of a neatly handled rake.

Billboards and store-bought signs were fewer; pieces of plywood painted white and hanging from a simple post-and-arm affair replaced them. In black hand lettering, the signs read CABINETMAKER, APPLE CIDER, BLACKSMITH, HANDMADE FURNITURE, EGGS, HOMEMADE BREAD AND HONEY, QUILTS, VEGETABLES. Most of the signs had a note at the bottom: NO SUNDAY SALES.

A black buggy, pulled by a leggy and spirited horse, bounded along the edge of the road.

I was softening up.

Then I got to the village of Intercourse.

Well, now. It wasn't that the village wasn't fine. In

fact, it was just what you'd hope for in a charming country village: a quilt shop, a candle barn, a couple of general stores, a post office, Brubaker's Garage, old oak and maple trees lining the street and (as all tourists learn), a hitching post out in front of the converted-to-computer bank.

What startled me were the Amish women; I'd never seen anything like them. White, stony faces, one after another along the sidewalks, in the general store, going in and out of the fabric shop. Each and every last one of them—girl or ancient—marched purposefully along, as if conscripted for duty. Each wore a massive black bonnet with a huge black bill that all but encircled her face and stuck out maybe an inch and a half from it. Most wore black shoes, black stockings, and a black cape worn over a black apron, which was worn over a black dress.

Not one smiled or so much as looked at me or anybody else. They had their eyes drilled into the sidewalk. All of their faces were very smooth, as if they'd never been broken in by laughing or kissing or crying. It was a wonder to me they would ever need a midwife.

Frankly, I didn't think I could deliver their babies. Midwifery is an intimate profession. In order for me to help a woman have her baby in the way that is easiest and healthiest for her, I have to see some of her interior composition—her physical and emotional strengths and weaknesses—and I need to see them quickly and surely. My whole manner—my touch, my words, my knowledge, my joking, my gossip, my instruction, and my silence—adjusts to her and to what I learn about her as we go along, and so each delivery is different since each woman has her own way to strength. The more a woman trusts her body and trusts me, the easier things are. The less obstructed the woman is, the less shielded she is from her body and from her emotions, the better her delivery.

That's why the births of those inner-city girls went so well. Being so young and so clearly in need of help, they *had* to trust us. They revealed themselves, gave up control, and allowed us to guide them to their bodies.

These Amish women—as cold, joyless, and ascetic as they seemed to be—would shield themselves from the intelligence of their bodies. Not only did they keep outsiders at a distance, but judging from their scarlike lips, they kept themselves at a distance too. You would probably have to use dynamite and a pickax to dislodge their babies.

I was glad I'd taken a half-holiday attitude toward this trip because the chance of my taking a job with Stephen Kaufman, doctor to the stony-faced women, was very slim. Not only would the deliveries be difficult and the babies reluctant to live, but I would have to spend my time with these dreary types. No thank you. Give me back my reggae mamas.

Still, I thought I would go ahead and talk to the doctor. No reason not to. I left the commercial roads and cut over to Paradise on farm roads.

The farms stopped me. They were perfect. They were absolutely exquisite. Each one was minutely cared for, as if the rows were pulled up straight each morning and the corners tucked in at nightfall. The soil was looser than at other farms; it was lighter, fluffed up, as if it had been given a good beating in a copper bowl.

I drove along a stream bed bounding with spring rains and watched where it widened into a pool by a farmhouse. Ducks sailed across the pond as if in serene possession of their affairs. I watched. There was no traffic and so few sounds. I rolled down the window and let the smell of the earth fill the car. I thought I could hear a duck paddling across the pond. I was awestruck.

I stared at the plowed earth, at the breathing, fertile soil all around me. And then I began to cry. After the assaults I had felt and seen in the cities, assaults of man against woman, woman against child; after the endless asphalted city floor; after the heavy metal-dust smell of power coursing along boulevards and into dark buildings, here—here, all this time, these people had been taking care of the soil.

I drove around a curve of a hillside. On it, a boy of ten or eleven years, barefoot on an unsaddled white mare, was riding up plowed rows. The horse pulled a plow and behind the plow, the boy's father walked. He carried a little girl on his back and stepped, barefooted also, up the rows of newly turned earth. I continued, afraid to breathe for fear of disturbing what I saw on the road to Dr. Kaufman's office.

Amish couples sat side by side in matching costumes in Dr. Kaufman's waiting room. In addition to their black pants, the men wore black coats with hook-and-eye closings. Their black, flat-brimmed hats hung from pegs by the door. The women had taken off their outdoor bonnets.

Here I need to explain something. Indoors, each woman wears a white organdy "covering," a gathered and banded cap that is shaped like a heart at the crown and covers the back of her head. It is secured to her hair with a straight pin, which is driven through a narrow band of organdy that runs across the top of her head and down either side. The combination of the straight pin and the severe stretching of the hair away from the center part often causes a pool of baldness at the top of a woman's head. That these women were able to secure their covering to the few thin remaining hairs seemed impossible to me at first. I was fascinated; I found myself studying the pins and bare skin and stray hairs the way a child studies the first deformed person they ever see. "What is that, Mama?" or, in this case, "Mama, does she put the pin in her skin?" Like the child, I was uncomfortable in seeing this unnatural arrangement, but more than anything, I was brazenly curious. I stared at every opportunity.

Just so you'll know, the caps are fastened without causing bleeding.

For more formal times, like going to the doctor, the Amish woman is sure to tie the ends of the bands of her covering not tightly under her chin, but loosely, so that a small white bow rests on her chest just below the hollow of her throat. The effect is sweet and virginal. When she's busy or just around the house, she often leaves the little bands running free, instead of tied, and they blow and play about her shoulders.

The Amish, Dr. Stephen Kaufman explained, were quiet and reserved around physicians, as they were around any English. They go to a doctor, it was glibly said, for "birth, death, and when they cut their hands off." Dr. Kaufman didn't know much about their beliefs, and, like a lot of people in the area, he thought of them as a simple, plain people without any education who, he observed, didn't always take his advice.

His idea was to build a bigger general practice

among the Amish by delivering more of their babies. A midwife was a way to increase his access to them and they seemed to like the idea, he said. I was to talk to some of his prenatal patients after he was done with them.

"Are you thinking of coming here?" Priscilla asked. She had no scar mouth. She had no captain's face, no infantryman's single-mindedness. Instead of black, she wore a bright blue dress. She smiled gaily, her face shone with eagerness. It seemed as if the idea of my coming was quite wonderful to her.

"Yes I am," I said and waited, wanting to get her purest response.

"Well," she said, "we'd be glad to have a woman to deliver our babies again. Dr. Kaufman is a good doctor, but it's different with a man. Men don't understand. Ever since Dr. Ruth had her accident, we've had to have men. And then some of us would like to have our babies at home. Dr. Kaufman said you might deliver babies at home."

And then she asked me if I knew how she could get her figure back again.

When I asked Stephen what he told the women about weight, he said, "I didn't think these women ever thought about things like that."

Men! I could certainly understand that these women got doughy and didn't like it. It was being a farmer's wife: too much cooking all the time and no one probably even bothered to explain about calories to them. It would be easy to help these women lose a few pounds.

We drove out to visit some patients.

Since it was Monday, we stepped under the weekly wash. In each and every farmyard the wash snapped on the lines in the same order: black pants from big to small; shirts—lawn green, sky blue, lavender—from big to small; dresses, the same; and then on to less distinguished items—shorts, socks, sheets, and dozens and dozens of diapers. Stephen warned me to be careful not to drive over the buggy shafts (the long poles that attach the horse to the buggy) either coming in or, more likely, backing out.

Each Amish kitchen we visited was immaculate. The floor, always of linoleum, shined back at us. The countertops were clear, the sink scrubbed, and all the dishes put away. The walls were painted green—the same color they used to have in hospitals—and the cupboards were pine. The kitchens were big—the center of virtually all activity in the house—and furnished with a big table in the center. There might be a couch and a chair too, but the table was the thing.

Children assembled willy-nilly at the corners of the room and stared wide-eyed at Dr. Kaufman and me. After a while a little one would break ranks and come over to his mother and crawl determinedly into her lap. The woman would talk quietly and cheerfully but without show. She would laugh and smile and stroke her children's hair. Shortly after we'd arrive, her husband would come in from the barns or fields, and pulling up another chair, he would talk with us too. They'd offer us ice cream, custard, cookies, and pretzels. We'd slow down and talk at a farmer's pace—with more space between words and ideas. I liked it; I remembered it from Westford Hill, Maine.

Over and over again I heard about Dr. Ruth, the woman who'd been doing home and hospital deliveries for the Amish for thirty years. She'd had an accident and ended up in a wheelchair, and the women were stuck. "Dr. Ruth was rough sometimes, she'd give the babies a hard pull sometimes, and she made mistakes," they told me, "but she was terrible busy and she worked hard. We feel she cared about us and our babies. She'd get us to the hospital if there was going to be a problem, like if there were going to be twins or something." Dr. Ruth delivered five thousand babies before she retired.

"Now we only have these other doctors—not Dr. Kaufman, but the other ones—and we're not sure they always handle things the best. My cousin had her labor start early—she was only seven months—but she was having contractions. She called the doctor. She and her husband, they thought maybe they should go to the hospital, but the doctor said that it was okay and he came out to her house and delivered the baby. It weighed just a little more than three pounds.

"My cousin and her husband, they wanted to know what to do about the baby after it was born because it was so tiny and they thought maybe they should go to the hospital with it. The doctor said just to put it in a box on the oven door and don't worry about it anymore."

The woman spoke softly, without rancor.

"Their baby died in the oven. And that was after the husband had carried the placenta out of the house to bury it. He found a second baby in the placenta, which the doctor had never bothered to check for or deliver. They had a hard time giving themselves up to that."

Stephen and I stumbled out of the house hearing that. We looked at each other in shock. Stephen said it made him ashamed of his profession and it made him think that sometimes it wasn't such a good idea that the Amish don't sue.

At the last house, the husband said to me, "Is it true that if you came here you would sit with the woman through her labor?"

VII ❧

Paradise Considered

I stayed two and a half days with Dr. Kaufman, talking, seeing the local hospital, and visiting patients. He showed me the rec center, set up an appointment for me with a real estate agent, explained about the school system if I should ever want to get married and have children. He showed me where the Chinese restaurants were. If I came, I would handle prenatal care office visits, I would labor-sit with the women at home and would deliver those babies too, although Dr. Kaufman would be present for the actual birth. He would handle hospital deliveries until such time as we were successful in getting me hospital privileges. Then I would be able to do midwife-attended hospital births and also follow home delivery patients into the delivery room in emergencies. He couldn't pay much, but we would renegotiate in a year, and besides it's cheap to live in the country.

Dr. Kaufman—Stephen, that is—was smart and he seemed to be trying to be a good doctor. He didn't know much about pregnancy—because he was a man, I suppose, and because in medical school they don't teach much about healthy, pregnant women. I thought I could do a good job for him, treat the women well, whether Amish or English. At the least, I could help protect the farm women from doctors who were killing their babies and I could teach them new ways, ways in which modern medicine could make their deliveries safer and more comfortable.

I drove home slowly along back roads, looking at farmhouses. These were country women; they cared about their gardens, their quilts, their children, and their homes. I understood them. I could give them good care.

What about Richie? I knew Richie was, without a doubt, the best of the males of the species, and besides, we had made what he called a "conscious decision" to live near each other. Richie had to fly; and after years of yearning and plotting, he got probably the only crew seat available to an old fellow—he was thirty-three—in the entire country. It was about an hour and a half from Lancaster County to the north Philly airport. That was too far. Maybe it wasn't. Maybe it would be all right. What of Richie really didn't want me to do this? What if he didn't want to move? What if we decided to live an hour and a half apart and I lost him?

Richie wasn't at his place when I got there. I let myself in, washed, scrubbed my face, changed my clothes. On the bureau I set a fresh-from-an-Amish-kitchen, molasses-based shoofly pie. Richie loved pie. There was a big white wicker rocker in the corner of his room, the kind with the high, peacock-tail back and wide woven arms. I'd gone out the week before and got a blue-and-white polka dot pillow for the seat of it; he said it was a waste of money and I thought it made things just right.

I wrapped myself in a blanket, rocked in the chair, and waited for Richie to come home. I looked at his shirts, lined up like a drill team marching blindly toward the closet wall, and at his shoes, toed up against the wall beneath his shirts. His books now included *Zorba the Greek*, Fritz Perls on *Gestalt Therapy*, as well as something like *The History of the Wing of the Airplane from the Sand Dunes at Kitty Hawk to the Salt Flats on the Mohave*, "with drawings of the major structural advancements." The books were arranged alphabetically by author along the top of his bureau. There was nothing hanging on the walls of the room except a narrow pine shelf that Richie had designed, built, and finished expressly to hold his grandfather's fiddle. It had been in his parents' attic in Island Falls, Maine, for years, then had gone astray. Richie, hearing that it was about to fall into unappreciative hands, made a special trip to Massachusetts to retrieve it. It rested securely now against the columbines and nasturtiums on the wallpaper of his room in this boardinghouse in suburban Philadelphia.

Richie and I had met—well, met wouldn't be the right word, more like exploded into each other's lives —at my parents' summer cabin on Pleasant Pond in northern Maine during that summer break from school in Glasgow. For three weeks, Richie and I spent our days paddling from cove to cove on Pleasant Pond; talking, swimming, picnicking, and visiting every last Maine character with a moving jaw—all of them Richie's friends. At night we curled up by the wood stove at his cabin and talked some more.

Richie'd grown up in Island Falls and had gotten a degree in engineering from the state university.

When I met him, all he'd seen of the world was Maine and parts of Vietnam; all he'd known of work was potatoes, sewer plant design, and runway construction. True, he did know how to fly, but he hadn't flown far, and the time had come, he said, to break out, to open up his consciousness, seek truth and all that. Richie'd worked up these ideas while reading *Siddhartha*, the *I Ching*, *Walden*, and *The Greening of America* in a construction trailer on the edge of the Frenchville runway. I was impressed.

He'd get up from his rocker, stir up the fire, walk out on the porch and kill a bat with his tennis racket, bring me a dish of ice cream, and one more time, he would laboriously explain that he did not want now, nor did he ever want, a dependent woman in his life. Never could abide them. And at the moment, he was plowing himself into his self-discovery business. He'd arranged a leave of absence from work and found just the car he'd been looking for; he had the route mapped out. He wanted to spend lots of time "standing around tumbleweed in Texas and," he said, "there's a place in California where you can sit in hot tubs that are cantilevered over the Pacific Ocean. Think of that, Penny. Not lobster shacks and death-cold winds, but hot tubs by the sea!"

After he'd finished up self-discovery, and if he could find somebody who could fit him with proper contact lenses, he was going to become a commercial pilot, or if that failed, he was going to Oman and make lots of money as an engineer.

Then and only then might he consider allowing a totally self-sufficient woman in his life.

Assiduously I went over my entire past for proof of my self-reliance. I told Richie how I'd navigated white water in the Sierras; had taken pregnant criminals on outings around California; had built a VW; put up all that weathered barn board in my farm in Maine; not to mention cooking, canning, sewing, and lambing. I mentioned how I had single-handedly put myself through a crash nursing program in Saint Louis, one of America's most dangerous cities. (I described in blood-chilling detail how I drove through the city one night with friends when I had the flu and had to throw up, but we all knew we could not stop the car for fear of being victims of random attack, so we continued driving through the streets, while I hung my head out the window, vomiting and thinking I would be lucky if no one took a pot shot at my head, hanging as it was like a tetherball from the car window.) Furthermore, I went on, I had endured the dismal and morally debilitating days in the male urology ward in Highlands General Hospital, and told him how, when I got my midwifery degree, I would plunge directly into Maine's remote parts and deliver babies all by myself.

I also told him about A. Robert Peterson, a contact lens magician I knew in California.

Richie reached over to me and pulled me close to him. He said the same words then that he would say when he put me on the plane to Scotland: "I just hope you are what you seem to be."

Since then I'd been trying.

By the time I'd finished my work in Glasgow, Richie had been west and back, and these days he talked to me, he helped me, he got a hot water bottle for my back when I had cramps, he put his arms around me and held me. He was funny, he certainly had no fear of teasing me, and he was always wandering off to places like Albuquerque in the back of a plane and then coming home to tell me absurd stories about how he was taken hostage by a gang of marauding women who wore yellow lipstick and lived in a cave deep in the shadow of the Grand Canyon, but loyal to the end, he'd won his escape by splitting their sides with stories of folks from Island Falls, Maine.

Richie wasn't perfect. For one thing, he was too organized—I had made more mess since I arrived at his place that afternoon that he had made in the six months previous. Furthermore, he was a man and probably couldn't be trusted. And finally, he couldn't understand why I got hysterical about some things. But I loved Richie.

Richie's room was only ten minutes from north Philly airport.

I started to think again about Lancaster County. My second day there, Stephen and I stopped at the home of a woman whose husband kept running away. (Actually, we had tried to visit the first day, but the yard had been filled with black buggies and Stephen said we shouldn't intrude.) Some Amish, even though they want to join the church and do, even though they get married and have their babies, can't stay within the community. I'm sure there are all kinds of reasons for running—all the ones that make those of us on the outside do it, plus some that are peculiar to the Amish culture.

Ike, Lydia's husband, was that way. They'd had their fourth baby and Ike had run away again, this time for so long that the Amish elders had to go to Boston to get him. He'd ended up at some church door, shaking and incoherent. Fortunately someone in the congregation knew about the Amish.

The elders brought him home, but he couldn't do his work and he was about to lose his milking cows for the lack of a decent roof on his barn. That first day when we drove by, the Amishmen from the neighborhood were crawling all over the barn roof; they had it finished by chore time. The women were inside making a meal for the thirty or so men who were working.

When Stephen and I saw Lydia, Stephen asked her how Ike was doing. She thought he was better. He was eating something and he'd slept the night before. In the time we talked, she never said a word against him; she never complained about the work and worry he caused her; she never said, "If he loved me, he wouldn't do this to me." She stayed at the farm, looked after their four babies, and waited for him to come home and to get better. She did wonder sometimes, she said, whether he should go someplace for help with his mental problems. But now that he was getting better, she didn't think of that so much.

Back in Richie's room, I sat in the wicker chair and watched the sky wash pink in behind the twigs and branches of the elm trees. For a while I thought about the pots and bottles I had in storage in Maine. I got up and had a piece of Richie's pie. Then I read for a long time, and dragging myself in my blanket, I curled up and went to sleep on Richie's bed. He didn't come home until much later; there had been some kind of delay in Boston.

In the morning I told him I wanted to go work with Dr. Kaufman.

He wanted to know how long this moving around was going to go on. Yes, he wanted an independent woman. Yes, he wanted me to have a career on my own. Yes, he admired me. But ever since he'd known me it was one stand after another. Maine, Saint Louis, Glasgow, Philadelphia, not to mention white-rapids riding in California, and now, of all places, Paradise, Pennsylvania. Perhaps I would never stop. We finally had a place where we could do the work each of us wanted to do, where we could be together, where we could make a home if we decided to, but no, I had to go a hundred miles out in the country, work for peanuts, and deliver babies at home, which, he reminded me, I had said was ethically unacceptable. "I don't suppose you remember throwing yourself against the wall and shrieking 'ethically unacceptable'?" he asked, licking his fingers and serving himself another piece of shoofly pie.

"Richie, I want you to come and see."

"I've seen cow manure."

"Please, Richie."

We drove out the next weekend in his 1965 VW Beetle, which had gaping joints and no heat. Richie had a cold; bitter winds and rain darkened the landscape and shriveled up our skin and bones. Richie drove with a blanket wrapped around his shoulders and blew his nose. He saw nothing that interested him. "A bunch of dirt farmers dressed up in Walt Disney costumes," he said.

I called Stephen Kaufman the following Monday morning and accepted the job. I didn't understand quite why I did it, but I did.

Three weeks later I delivered my first baby at home.

I was overwhelmed with the responsibility. I'd delivered a lot of babies by then; that is, enough to know that things went wrong. That was my job—knowing about things that went wrong. As a midwife, I could help a good, healthy birth be a relatively comfortable and probably a richer experience for a mother, but by and large, she could do it by herself with her husband or a friend. What she needed me for was to anticipate problems and to handle emergencies. By the number of them I'd seen, I had no trouble justifying my presence at a birth.

At Booth, I had backup: not only fetal monitors, intrauterine pressure monitors, X-ray machines, ultrasound scans, suction, oxygen, drugs, IVs, blood transfusions, but also anesthesiologists, obstetricians, surgeons, neonatologists, and skilled nurses, not to mention a scrub basin and a sterile trolley.

But what do you do about emergencies when you're standing in somebody's bedroom in a farmhouse in the middle of a cornfield, in a place where the fanciest technology is hot and cold running water and your medical team is comprised of a farmer who —at best—had delivered his own calves.

Take flat babies. They have poor color—that is, they are blue or gray and their bodies are limp; they show little or no enthusiasm about breathing. It was my clear impression that most babies were flat. In the hospital you automatically cleaned out air passages with a suction tube that's piped right into the room; then, without breaking rhythm, you leaned in the other direction and grabbed for an oxygen mask so you could, if necessary, "bag" the baby, that is, pump oxygen into its lungs. You could stimulate its heart. You could turn to the neonatologist and have him or her take the problem off your hands, especially if the mother was having difficulty.

Suppose Stephen was late for a delivery, the baby was flat, and the mother started to hemorrhage? How would I resuscitate the baby, keep the father from fainting, get the emergency team on the road, and stop the hemorrhaging all at the same time? And how long does it really take for one of these country emergency teams to respond to a call? Women die in childbirth, for heaven's sake. If the placenta breaks away from the uterine wall in just the right place at just the right time, a woman can loose enough blood in fifteen minutes to die.

And I was off to deliver babies where there might not be any electricity and the nearest phone was either in the chicken coop or across the pasture.

My first delivery was in an Amish cottage, fenced in with an honest-to-goodness white picket fence. I turned into the drive just as Enos, the father, was tucking his two-year-old onto the seat of an open buggy. Enos—with dark wavy black hair, a square jaw, eyes the color of a mountain stream, six feet tall and broad-shouldered; in other words, a picture-book husband—waved, grinned, and said he'd be right back. He prompted his horse and pulled off down the gravel drive to take little Johnny, the two-year-old, to his aunt's house.

Thinking I would find Katie stretched out in her bed, I turned to go up the steps to the back porch. Just then she popped out the back door. She had a paintbrush in her hand.

"Oh," she said, "hi. Oh, my goodness, I'm not quite ready. I was putting the final coat of lacquer on this rocking chair when I started to have stronger contractions. I just wanted so much for it to be done, so I could rock the baby in it.

"Then I decided that I'd better call Enos. He works out at the machine shop, so I went to the neighbor's phone, and I didn't want to call you because they'd know, but I just called Enos and said I thought he ought to come home."

She'd cleaned the brush and now she laid it down on some neatly folded newspapers spread out on a corner of the porch. Not only did the rocker look freshly lacquered, but it appeared that the porch floor had been scrubbed and waxed not long ago. She stopped talking for a moment when she stood up, put her hands on her hips, and stretched out her back.

"Is that a contraction?" I asked.

"Yes it is."

"Is it pretty strong?"

"Yes, I believe it is, and I haven't put that plastic thing on the bed yet."

We walked through an immaculate kitchen and a spotless living room. She'd gotten her husband off to work, gotten her toddler up, washed, fed, and dressed, cleaned up the breakfast dishes, straightened up the living room, and painted a rocking chair. I think it was about 8:30 in the morning.

I had my small bag in my hand.

"Before we make the bed, let's see how dilated you are." I was thinking that this woman couldn't be too far along since she was running around like she was getting ready for her first date.

Wrong. Nine centimeters.

"Where's that plastic sheet?" I said. "Looks to me like you're about to have a baby."

She chattered her way off to the linen closet and back. "Oh, I'm so excited," she said. "I can hardly wait. Every night when I go to bed, I say to Enos, 'Maybe tonight I'll have the baby. Maybe by tomorrow morning it will be lying right here between us.' And then in the morning when I wake up, I'm so disappointed because it didn't happen and I've been thinking I would have to wait all the way until the next night before there was even a chance again. I never even thought I could have it during the day. Enos keeps telling me not to be so impatient. He says he has to remind me that he believes the baby really will be born."

She stopped again for another contraction, and as soon as it passed she went back to spreading out the plastic sheet over the mattress cover. I was supposed to be helping her, but I had trouble concentrating. I kept staring. The woman was nine centimeters dilated and she was bustling about furiously.

We finished making up the bed, then she thought maybe she'd change from her dress into a gown. Next thing I knew, she'd hopped onto the bed. Her face was flushed and she was ready to push.

Stephen's office was only a quarter of a mile away. I'd put a call in to him on my radio as soon as I checked Katie that first time, and he pulled in just as she was getting serious about pushing her baby out. Enos followed right behind him. He went to Katie's side and grabbed her hand.

The three of us attended quietly. A couple of times Katie said it hurt and she called her husband's name, and he got closer to her and held her so she could push more easily.

The baby, a boy, popped out as if he were on his way to the outfield to catch a long fly. I put him on the bed at Katie's side, and she curled herself around him.

"Oh," she said, "look at him. Look at our new baby. Oh, I wonder what Johnny will think."

Enos stroked her head and said, "So now you have your baby."

And she said, "Oh, my, look how beautiful he is. Just look. Oh, Enos, I love him already."

I checked Katie to see if there were any tears in

her perineum. There weren't. For a moment Stephen stood back with his arms folded and watched. "I couldn't have done it like that," he said to me and then he went on to check the baby. In a few minutes, he left, giving me responsibility for the after care.

I cleaned Katie up, washed the baby at the kitchen sink, and got him started at his mother's breast. Then I went out into the kitchen to give them a chance to be alone and to do my paperwork.

Pretty soon Enos came out, opened the desk, and started riffling through papers. He pulled one out, looked at me, and smiled peacefully. "I never want to choose a name before the baby's born," he said. "I write down a list of names that I think of, but then I wait until I see the baby before I choose one. No reason," he said softly, leaving time between his words the way these people do, "it's just my way."

I went back into the bedroom just as Enos was getting ready to go back down the road for little Johnny. A buggy was passing by and you could hear it slow down as it came near the house. "Oh, I know who that is," Katie said. "It's my sister. We were supposed to go together to our appointments at Dr. Kaufman's today. I guess she'll be surprised I don't go with her. I guess Enos will tell her how come I'll stay at home today. Oh, I hope she stops by on her way back from the doctor."

I was staring again. This was not a hyperactive person, just a cheerful, enthusiastic young mother. But she'd just had a baby and she was still full of energy. Next thing I know, she says, "Can I get up? Just for a minute. I just have to try something. I just need to go in the other room."

I couldn't think of a reason to say no, but, then, I was pretty stunned at the time. I helped her stand, made sure she wasn't feeling dizzy, and watched her go to a bureau in the second bedroom. She came back with a tiny white baby cap.

"I just have to see how he'll look in this. I made it for him and I just can't wait to see him in it." She plunked herself down on the bed and picked the baby up. The baby, now a good forty-five minutes old, went into her lap and she busily put the little bonnet on him. "It fits perfectly," she said. "Look at him, look at our baby."

I waited until Enos returned and then left. A buggy was coming from the direction of Dr. Kaufman's office. I waved as I passed by and they smiled and waved back.

I was totally bewildered. And euphoric. I'd never seen a birth quite like this one.

VIII

Spring Road

"Penny speaking."

"Is this Penny?"

"Yes, this is Penny."

"The wife, she has a pain."

"What fer pain is that?"

"Why, it's the pain down low."

"Does it come and go?"

"Yah."

"Is it time for me to come?"

"Whatever you think."

"Who would this be?"

"Elam Stoltzfus."

"Oh, would your wife be Mary over on School Road, then?"

I quickly learned the way to ask questions and to identify people, but it took me a long time to get used to phone calls from Amish fathers-to-be. They just didn't seem to want to tell much. In the first place, an Amishman isn't likely to go in for much detail when talking with outsiders. But put him on the phone and he'll clam up even more; he's not used to it. After I'd been in the community for a while, I got a letter from an Amishwoman that helped me understand the whole thing. She wanted to thank me for something, but she explained that she had never learned to enjoy the phone—mainly because she never used it much —and besides, she was afraid the person on the other end couldn't understand her.

If you're going to be nervous that your message won't get across when you're making a thank-you phone call, you're likely to be in real difficulty when you have to call somebody up and hope they understand you need them to come deliver your baby. And if that isn't enough, this Amish husband is standing in a phone shed, his wife is at least a quarter of a mile away, and I start asking questions he doesn't know the answer to, like how far apart the contractions are and "what fer else" would I want to know anyway. What he does know is that he's scared the baby's going to come roaring out of the channel before I get there to catch it. All of these things make him forget that his wife may not be the only woman in Lancaster County due to have a baby.

Not that I hadn't been waiting for the call from Elam Stoltzfus. Only a few days before I had been with Elam and Mary Stoltzfus in Stephen's office. We sat with our hands folded reasonably in our laps and decided what to do when Mary went into labor. She was likely to be early and by as much as three weeks; she always was, they told me. It always went fast but smoothly, and she wanted to have this baby at home. Stephen got up, walked casually over to the window, looked out for a moment, turned around, leaned loosely against the wall, slipped his hands in his pockets casually the way doctors do when they're trying to tell you that some things that seem like life and death to the rest of us mortals are nothing at all to be concerned about.

"I can't think why you shouldn't have this baby at home," he said.

I can, I said to myself, unable to conceive of doing a home delivery unless conditions were textbook perfect.

What about the special risks of prematurity, Doc? I wanted to say. What about hypothermia? The baby might not stay warm enough (preemies don't have enough body fat to keep them warm). And what about Respiratory Distress Syndrome? ("Get the baby to special care," is what the midwife's texts read.) And that was just for starters.

"There are, of course, some risks associated with prematurity," Dr. Kaufman went on, "specifically hypothermia and Respiratory Distress Syndrome..."

Mary and Elan listened and nodded thoughtfully. Mary was quiet, dark-eyed, soft-spoken, and dutiful. She wouldn't panic; Mary wasn't the type to panic, I said to myself, anticipating the direction of this discussion. Mary's already had three babies. She probably delivers leaning against the wall with her hands slipped casually in her pockets. And her husband— take one look at him and you'd know everything was going to be all right. He appeared to be one of those men who could fix anything, make anything work— the type who could milk a cow and paint the barn at the same time. His children probably came out singing "John Henry, he could hammer..."

"But these are unlikely to occur and I believe we are well equipped to handle them if they do," he concluded.

Mary and Elam looked at each other for a moment

and then Elam said, "I believe we'll have our baby at home, then." That was all. It was settled.

Naturally, I didn't sleep after that. Besides going over in my mind the subtleties of delivering a premature child, I had to stay awake to test my radio every five minutes.

The plan was that Elam would call me first, I would call Stephen, and we'd both go over to Mary's; but I would get there first because I was closer. I had memorized and practiced the route; I figured seven minutes. This was Mary's fourth baby; the last one had come in three hours—this one wasn't likely to take much longer.

The night the call came was bitter cold; ice crept all over the roads. I hadn't planned on icy roads in late April. It took me about fifteen minutes to get to Mary's house, instead of seven.

My headlights flickered on the ice that had formed on the gravel in the drive. Elam came to the door, poker in his hand. Thinking it was going to be a normal spring night, he'd let the stove die way down, and when I got there at about 3:30 A.M. he was stoking it up. He apologized.

The kitchen was starting to warm up, but the bedroom—way in the back corner of the house—was still freezing. Walking through the dark hallways to the bedroom, I prayed for time; but after one look at Mary I gave that up. This baby was waiting neither for warmer weather nor for Dr. Easy Does It.

I had on my down vest and long johns and so I stopped noticing the cold quickly enough. As for Mary, well, you can't be cold when you're pushing out a baby; it's impossible. And I suppose we managed to keep Elam running back and forth for one thing and another so that he stayed warm. Anyway, by the time baby Joel's brow showed, we had all forgotten how awfully cold it was in that bedroom.

Until his little body followed. He weighed only five and a half pounds and as I lifted him and went to set him on his mother's stomach, I saw steam rising from his body like breath from a horse's nostrils in the dead of winter.

I threw a blanket over him, reached under it, clamped and cut the cord in one move, bundled him, and handed him to his father. "You go downstairs and you hold this baby over the stove." Elam smiled, put his giant farmer's paw under the wee bundle, stuffed it affectionately in the corner of his arm, and started out toward the kitchen. "It is very important for the baby to stay warm," I said with great firmness.

I heard no crunching of the gravel, saw no headlights through the bedroom window. Dr. Kaufman was nowhere to be seen.

I stayed with Mary to deliver the afterbirth, got rid of the wet and bloody sheets, wrapped them up, washed her, helped her change her gown, tucked the blankets up under her chin and went downstairs to find Elam and the baby. It had been about twenty minutes.

I'll never forget the sight in that kitchen. Everything was in order, as usual. There was the kerosene lantern going on the kitchen table. Elam was standing in the middle of the kitchen in the halo of warm light, a grin on his face, sweat pouring down his face in a stream, his arms outstretched straight over the coal stove, and the wee baby in his hands above it, like a blessed offering.

"I guess if he's warm as me, he'd be warm enough" was all he said.

Dr. Kaufman's car had skidded on the ice and he got stuck for a while in a ditch. He came in about the time the back bedroom began to warm up.

Joel's four now and thriving.

IX

The Country Hospital

By *telling* you about Mary and Elam and how Stephen didn't make it until after their baby was born, I'm afraid I might be giving you the wrong impression of him. As I said, Stephen is a fine doctor. His decision to do the delivery at home was a sound one and his not getting there in time was just one of those things that happens in a rural practice. We skid on ice, get stuck in snowbanks, our beepers go haywire, we drop our supply of sterile gloves on the path leading up to a house.

Take, for instance, another delivery, on another freezing night, that became nothing less than a series of emergencies. The mother, whom I had carefully interviewed in my office, chose the last minute to remember to reveal to me that she hemorrhaged after her births. She waited for just a second or two to let that sink in and then she delivered a baby who didn't want to start breathing. I called the ambulance, and though fearing the mother might start to bleed at any moment, I had to begin working on resuscitating the baby. I carried him to a spot near the stove. Like that night at Elam and Mary's, I had on my down jacket, only in this case I had it on simply because I hadn't had a chance to take it off.

So I kneeled in front of the stove, sweat pouring off my body the way sweat poured off Elam's, breathing for the baby, and every now and then skipping a beat to call into the other room, "Is she bleeding at all?" She wasn't.

This went on for about seven minutes, until the emergency crew arrived. I didn't have to call in to the other room anymore, but I did have to go on breathing for the baby for another thirteen minutes.

The little fellow, so long pleaded with, so long breathed for, was finally convinced to join us, and he then took vigorous hold. Within minutes he was pink and warm; his reflexes were excellent. We relaxed for about thirty seconds, everyone rejoiced about the baby's liveliness, then I waved off the emergency crew, reached into my bag for a prefilled Pitocin syringe so I could give the poor mother a shot and she could more quickly deliver her afterbirth. The Pitocin, having been out in my car under the icy sky, was frozen solid. No matter, I thought. I would simply put the syringe on the stove for a moments to melt the liquid inside while I went over to check the mother.

I put the syringe on the corner of the stove, went into the other room to the mother, felt her uterus, talked to her for a few moments, and by the time I got back to the syringe it had been transformed into a molten, bubbling puddle on top of the stove.

That's the sort of mistake that teaches us to be humble in our work.

I was able to stimulate the uterus by massaging it from the outside, and she delivered the placenta with no difficulty, although more slowly than she would have with the Pitocin.

As we were cleaning up I asked her why she supposed she hadn't hemorrhaged.

"It's simple," she said with downcast eyes. "I was too scared."

Stephen was a genuine ally.

When I accepted the job with him, we agreed that I would immediately apply for hospital privileges, that he would sponsor my application and energetically support it. We both knew there would be opposition from the other doctors, but we also felt it could be managed.

Getting privileges was important to me. I had told Stephen that I had no great desire to do home births. "Every single baby," I said with great conviction, "deserves optimal birth conditions." At the time, I felt strongly that a hospital was more likely to provide those conditions.

I must say that after I knew Country Hospital* better, I was less absolute. I hadn't practiced in a level-one hospital, like Country Hospital, before coming to Lancaster County and so I didn't fully appreciate their limitations. Designed to serve rural areas, level-one hospitals are equipped to give only the most basic care. They tend to have more general specialists working in them: internists or cardiologists. An important part of their expertise is in emergency intervention and referral.

---

*I want to remind the reader that I've invented the name of this and every other hospital in the book except for Booth. I've also changed the names of places and, with the exceptions mentioned in the preface, people's names. I have no interest in exposing a particular institution, because I don't believe individual institutions are the issue; the issue is a philosophy and style of care that is, in my experience, found in many hospitals today.

* * *

At Country Hospital, then, there was a room for delivery and there was one for surgery; there were nurses, needles, and telephones. They did have a fetal monitor, a gift from a local benefactor, but no one knew how to use it, so it was parked in a remote basement closet with its plastic cover still on. There was no intensive care nursery, no pediatrician, no obstetrician, no neonatal specialist. If a baby was in danger, you had to rush him or her to the level-two hospital, Infants and Childrens Hospital, fifty minutes away.

The big advantage to having a maternity patient in Country Hospital, from what I could tell, was that she was closer to emergency surgery, should it be needed. That and the fact that, for the professional, the hospital is a reassuring, supportive environment; you are surrounded by a system that has been invented to help you give care. If I were, for example, to do something reckless like rest a plastic syringe of Pitocin on a hot radiator, there would not only be other syringes of Pitocin to replace it, but there would be someone to go for them and someone to clean up after me.

Anyway, I wanted to do midwife-attended hospital deliveries and I wanted to be able to stay with home birth patients who, in an emergency, might have to be transported through the surgery doors—a barrier I couldn't cross without privileges.

So immediately after I arrived in Paradise, we made our application and they—that is, some of the doctors—began their resistance.

Stephen threw himself into our side of the effort. He got himself seated on the proper committees. He showed them data proving that midwives are good for babies and mothers. I don't remember exactly what evidence we chose to include, but it's likely we cited a rural Madera County, California, project in which the death rate for newborns dropped by more than half when nurse-midwives practiced. We educated, we wrote letters, and we answered questions. We documented my education, training, licensure, and skills. Stephen took his colleagues to lunch. He put on a gigantic poolside party (complete with a cameo appearance by the highly respected Dr. Ruth in her wheelchair), so that the doctors and their wives could meet me in pleasant surroundings.

After five months of effort, we succeeded in getting a resolution passed that gave me privileges to practice in the hospital as an "allied health professional." We went out to dinner to celebrate.

And the next morning we read the newspaper account: "Midwife Joins Hospital Staff, Five Doctors Quit." That is, they gave up their staff privileges; they refused to work in a hospital that allowed me to work. One of the physicians was quoted as saying that he just felt the decision was "a step backward." He implied that care from a midwife was lower-quality care, that it was somewhat primitive.

Now that was absurd. Aggravating and infuriating too. But basically absurd. Of all the arguments one might level at midwifery, that one, applied as it was to the nurse-midwife practicing in a hospital setting, is poorest. Think about it: the hospital is there and the doctor is just down the hallway. The midwife, an expert in normal labor and delivery, stays by the mother's side for the course of labor the way a nurse can't (the nurse has half a floor to patrol), and the way a doctor can't (the doctor's overhead would never allow it and, besides, it's a waste of skills). If anything looks irregular, the midwife can push a button and all the high-tech intervention available can come rolling in the door.

But he said it, and, of course, everybody started to wonder if maybe it's true: maybe midwives are a throwback; maybe they practice with hangers and fishhooks; maybe they do wear layers of petticoats that they never change. Oh, they might tear them up occasionally and stuff a strip or two into a mother's mouth to keep her quiet, but they don't take them off, wash them, and hang them in the sun to dry. Have you heard that midwives never pare their fingernails except into cauldrons of swamp brew?

I lost my temper.

In calmer moments, I understood the doctor to be saying that midwives were not highly trained enough to orchestrate the array of machinery and drugs that were necessary, in his opinion, to deliver babies.

We had to try to answer the challenge—that midwifery was lesser care—even though we knew it meant beating through a tangle of misconceptions about women, medicine, and childbirth. We now understood that our statistical demonstration that the midwife-attended childbirth was healthier for the mother (not to mention less costly) was wholly insufficient. The resistance to midwifery was more than a century deep; it went back to when science and technology were first applied to health care.

Let me explain. It used to be that midwives—female midwives—attended births. Their training was informal, that is, handed down from midwife to midwife and learned through experience. Their therapies were herbs, their interventions during labor were walking, positioning, massaging, and perhaps bathing.

Then, in a development independent of midwifery,

came the application of science and technology to the healing arts. Then came modern medicine, and with it the rise of physicians in a profession dominated by men. Medicine and male physicians gradually engulfed midwifery.

The overtaking was gradual, of course, and if you dip into the past, you'll find times when female midwives had more patients than male physicians and times when things were in balance. There was even a period when American doctors were advocating the kind of system Dr. Kaufman and I wanted to install at Country Hospital in the 1970s.

> From 1750 to approximately 1810 American doctors conceived of the new midwifery as an enterprise to be shared between themselves and trained midwives. Since doctors during most of that period were few in number, their plan was reasonable and humanitarian and also reflected their belief that, in most cases, natural processes were adequate and the need for skilled intervention limited, though important. Doctors therefore envisaged an arrangement whereby trained midwives would attend normal deliveries and doctors would be called to difficult ones.*

That didn't come to pass. Instead, we Americans became more enamored of technology and we American women, for complex reasons, became more passive in childbirth. Male doctors started taking all their tools and tricks, including forceps and cesarean sections, and applying them liberally (under the name of

---

* Richard W. and Dorothy C. Wertz, *Lying In: A History of Childbirth in America* (New York: The Free Press, a Division of Macmillan Inc., 1977), p. 44.

advancement) to passive women—made more malleable by the introduction of anesthesia.

Americans, more than people in other cultures, were enamored of technology and intervention in childbirth, and we got in the habit of intervening so much that the natural birth process became masked and we, the whole society, began to think of "birth as a potential disease."* When that doctor at Country Hospital "just felt" that midwifery represented a lower level of care, he was expressing a commonly held belief. He, and much of the rest of America, treat birth as if it were pathogenic, that is, as if something were wrong, as if it required corrective action, not to mention rescue. And, of course, midwives are not doctors.

Stephen Kaufman and I tried to explain that midwives attended normal births, that a major part of their professional training was in learning to screen out high-risk patients, and that they always had doctors backing them up. By demonstration, by articulation, and by our patience, we tried to explain.

At least we could tackle that doctor's objections; it had some substance buried in it. The other arguments just wore us down. Another doctor was quoted as saying that he objected to the decision because of some procedural flaw in the decision-making process; and another implied that you only used midwives when you didn't have enough doctors.

Stephen stayed with the effort, soothing, talking, educating. In newspaper interviews he spoke politely and patiently. He explained that many physicians hadn't had the opportunity to understand nurse-mid-

*Ibid., p. 236.

wifery, or other allied health professionals, for that matter. He said he felt that once they had some first-hand experience they would accept these other professionals and find their skills useful.

Meanwhile, I tried to do my part. I remained well groomed, cheerful, and professional; I answered all the questions the newspaper reporters asked me, factually, pleasantly, and simply. I explained that doctors and midwives did do things differently—that we were more likely to have a woman up and moving around during labor; that we would give her something to eat; that we were less likely to use medication and technology; and that we were less likely to cut the opening of the birth canal. Instead, we worked the tissue and stretched it.

I worked in the hospital. I behaved. I was quiet and unobtrusive in my practice. They gave me a small room for natural childbirth and they allowed my women to walk the halls and let me give them something light to eat so they could keep their energy up. I didn't do shaves and enemas routinely, I did fewer episiotomies than doctors, and I was delighted not to hook women up to the machinery because it prevented them from walking around and that helps keep a labor moving along.

Both Stephen and I believed that if we did a good job, if we were reliable, if we didn't make much of a scene, then the hospital and its doctors would realize we meant no harm and midwives could, with appropriate intervention by physicians, give mothers excellent care. We believed that women would actually be attracted to Country Hospital because it had midwifery services.

But the resistance held. One of Stephen's colleagues virtually abandoned his practice so he could devote full time to the cause. He filled a briefcase with midwife horror stories and stood at the front door of the hospital and handed them out as the doctors came in to work.

And the more I thought about it, the more peculiar the resistance seemed to me.

After all, Country Hospital was not a high-tech, high-intervention hospital. It was unusually simple and probably because of the people it served. A great many of the people who used Country Hospital were Mennonite families; certainly, Mennonite farm women dominated the labor and delivery patients.

Some of the doctors were Mennonite too, and they seemed to be less enamored of technology and more humble about their own skills. One of my most vivid memories in that hospital was watching one particular Mennonite surgeon prepare to perform a cesarean section. He would, each time before he cut, lift his scalpel—delicate instrument that it is, capable of saving the baby and mother, capable also of cutting a wound across the face of the unborn child—and hold it for a moment, poised on the tips of his thumb and forefinger. He regarded it ritually before he dropped his hand to cut. I liked to think he was investing the scalpel with a prayer.

I was working in a hospital where technology and intervention were not dominant; where the habits were not to overanesthetize, not to overcut, not to overdoctor women at childbirth. Yet even here, the doctors were foaming like mad dogs because a midwife was delivering babies.

That five doctors quit the hospital just to protest my practice surprised me, and then, as months went by and I deliveried babies quietly and healthily and still the battle raged, I began to realize that the reaction to my presence was far greater than the apparent threat. This was not a thoughtful acting out of society's debate on intervention and quality of care. This went to the root.

I believe now that many male doctors simply did not want a woman, especially a nondoctor, doing life-and-death work. By my success in giving good care, I was regularly showing that the doctors' knowledge was not sacred knowledge, that it was not inscrutable to all but the high priesthood of physicians.

Then, too, I was taking fees they thought should have been theirs. And finally, I was taking from them the power to control women who were having babies.

I remember talking to one doctor at Stephen's poolside party. A charming talker and a literate man, he loved especially to talk about himself. "From the moment we enter medical school," he said, "we are trained to think we are gods."

X

In the Fields

When I first moved to Lancaster County, I camped
out in an apartment. I threw a mattress on the floor
and slept in a snarl of bedclothes. I swam laps at the
rec center every day to keep my nerves from igniting,
and then rushed to the whirlpool. Usually I had the
little whirlpool room to myself and I'd turn the power
on to dynamo strength, take a deep breath, and dive
into a tuck at the bottom of the small plastic tub,
where I vanished for a merciful forty-five seconds
into a warm, pulsing, pounding, rolling, tingling vor-
tex of nothingness. In the beginning in Lancaster,
while I was on trial for a murder they were hoping I
would commit, I had to calculate and recalculate
every action, every decision, every attitude, twitch,
and gesture of my body and face. My sanctuary was
one minute of oblivion in a swirl of shooting bubbles.

Richie came to see me. He never said anything
more about my leaving Philadelphia, and in fact, I'm

not even sure he thought about it anymore. We were both shocked by what I'd done. Shocked and sobered.

We had thought we were only talking dreams, talking as lovers, we had thought our conversation flowed because of finding each other, we had thought we were suspending disbelief. Why should we, away from one another, opening the car door, sending away applications, or putting away the silverware, be convinced that I would stay with my enraptured vision of working as a midwife?

When I drove out to Lancaster County that first time, I should have known better. It was clear to me that my being a midwife for these people had always been true; this part of my life had been waiting for me. All the suspense, the anticipation, the agonizing decisions, the wondering if I was going to make it, had been mere accompaniments, diversions, and embellishments, which distracted me and made me believe I had some choice in the matter, when in fact I had none. Quite simply, I had come home.

I believe Richie felt it, too. When he eventually came out to find me, to figure out how to share a life with me under these circumstances, he was conceding humbly to an absolute.

It couldn't have been that easy for him, making the adjustment. He hadn't wanted any change, and now here I was putting every morsel of my being into thinking of how to handle the problems of home deliveries, into keeping calm and behaving while I was at the hospital, and into planning strategies to win over infuriated doctors. That didn't leave much of me for him.

Yet, within a few weeks he began looking for places to live between the airport at north Philly and the delivery room at Country Hospital. When he grew tired of hunting for rooms, he'd come and see me.

Sometimes I took him with me on house calls. I got him used to following buggies on the road and to the point where he, like me, began to hope one would appear in front of us and we'd be forced, like the buggy passengers, to go slow and look out the window.

One house in particular fascinated me. It was a regular two-story farmhouse with a broad low porch across the front and a massive oak tree spreading protectively over the front yard. The first time I passed the house I saw a bent, skeletal figure in the yard. She stood so still as to seem hung in the air beneath the tree. She wore a bonnet and an Amishwoman's dress, but was so frail that her body seemed to be of neither sex.

Unlike all other Amish farmhouses, which gleam with fresh white paint, hers was gray. Instead of the usual crisp green garden chairs on the front porch, there was a couch with humps on it where springs were breaking through. The outbuildings were covered with tar paper instead of white siding.

I made a point to go by the house whenever I could. Obviously the woman who lived there was ill and poor, but there was something about the house that made it different. It haunted me, but not in a bad way. I was drawn to it as if something special and good were there.

I eventually realized it was the way the place was kept. The lawn, balding though it was, was trimmed crisply each week; its edges were barbered like any prosperous lawn. The tar paper on the outbuildings was patched in squares, each one nailed neatly into place; there were no ragged edges flying in the wind.

The small garden was maintained. The window shades were drawn evenly each morning. The place was immaculate.

On these roads, apparently, poverty failed to poison either dignity or responsibility. Here one tended the little that one might have with as much discipline and order as one tended the much that one might have. Being stewards of the earth—as the Amish say they are—apparently meant being a steward of any part thereof, however great or small. Of course, the woman couldn't have done the work herself. Her family and her neighbors must have done it.

I drove Richie by that house.

During the first summer months that I was in the County, Richie and I would drive during the day and then, when the sky turned its usual, amazing moth-wing pink, we'd go for a walk through the covered bridge to an old stone mill. We'd sit and listen to the water slip by and wait for the legions of fireflies to arise, court, and bedazzle one another among the rushes.

Then we'd go home and eat roast chicken. I'd got into the habit of roasting a chicken for Richie. Elmer Ebersol started that.

One of our first times out, I took Richie over to make a house call on Elmer's wife, figuring that he would want to kill a chicken for us. Elmer was happy with the way his wife was treated before his baby was born and to show it he had started bringing me a chicken every time he brought her in for an appointment. In the last month before she delivered, I'd stop by the house to check her—it was too long a ride in a buggy to our office for a woman eight months pregnant—and sure enough, Elmer would put aside what he was doing and go out and get me a chicken while I waited.

I had barely pulled in the driveway and introduced my friend Richard Armstrong when Elmer, Amish romantic, said he thought I might want to roast a chicken for my friend the airline pilot. There was more than a hint there that if I did that up right, Richie might be willing to marry me.

"Would you like me to kill you a chicken?"

"If you'll let me give you a hand," said Richie, who knew how to be well mannered on a farm.

Elmer leaned against the car. "You sure you want to?" he said, looking at the city slicker and letting a slow smile unfold over his face.

"Why, yes. I believe I would," said Richie, getting more laconic by the word.

"A lot of folks lose their interest in eating chickens after they've seen one killed," Elmer said.

"I guess I'll take my chances," said Richie, and we followed Elmer into the house so that he could tell his wife to get the water boiling. At Elmer's house, the chicken-killing chores are divided up this way: Elmer's wife boils the water, gets instructions from the midwife on how to tend to the new baby, and keeps the older children occupied by allowing them to crawl all over the back of the sofa to the window-sill, where they can see kittens playing outside in the tree. Elmer's mother, Elizabeth, called Lizzie, comes over from her adjoining house. Lizzie makes the decisions on chicken-killing matters and she also cleans the chickens. Elmer catches the chicken, drops the hatchet on its neck, and does anything else he's told.

Richie and Elmer disappeared outside, and pretty soon Elmer came back in, saying that they'd captured the chicken and didn't I want to see Richie tying it up? I could tell I was supposed to be the audience of this affair, so I went, to see Richie putting the last bow knot in the legs of the chicken.

It's hard not to love a man who can catch and bind a chicken.

Next thing I know, Elmer picks up the stunned chicken and lays its bitty white neck right between two ordinary nails hammered into a log. Thwock.

The head went to one side and the body of the chicken, blood spurting out of its neck, to the other. Its wings flapped, it ran around, and the bloody fountain gushed while Richie and Elmer calmly talked. I turned my back and walked around the farmyard for a few minutes. Make of it what you will, I do not care for the sight of blood. Elmer went on talking about how his mother was an expert with chickens. She'd been gutting them since she was a child; the family used to make part of their living that way. They'd load their chickens on the back of a wagon and drive it right through Intercourse, selling chickens off the back as they went.

Couldn't do that anymore, that's for sure. So many regulations about refrigeration. A farmer couldn't afford to keep up with those regulations.

Lizzie had come out by then and she sent Elmer to fetch the boiling water, which he did. She told him to pour it into the tub and he did, and then she dunked the chicken into the scalding water.

I remembered that smell pretty well from when I was a kid, and I guess Richie must have, too, but neither one of us said a word. We both bent down and started pulling off feathers in hunks. When that was done, we backed off. Lizzie did the innards.

She pulled out the windpipe, careful to cut it clean at the bottom first; then she scraped off that gland at the tail—she wasn't sure what it was or why the chicken pecked at it, but her dad had told her to cut that off right away, so she always did. She was careful in handling the stomach; if you were careful, she said, you could pull out the lining of the stomach and its contents all in one fell swoop and that was more pleasant for everybody. "Do be careful to cut out the place where the throat tube connects to the stomach," she went on. "A lot of people get upset when they recognize a hole in something they're eating."

I tried to show enthusiasm for the gizzard and the heart and the lining of the stomach; I even initiated a search through the entrails to find a missing lung, which Lizzie wished to comment on. Then we rinsed the whole thing off and Lizzie directed Richie and Elmer to go off and bury the entrails in the yard.

The Ebersol family scurried about, gathering up corn, pole beans, lettuce, and cantaloupe to go with our roaster, and then they stood around in the farmyard—old Lizzie, Elmer and his wife, each one with a baby in their arms—and waved us off.

Richie used to say that going around with me was like being a groupie. It's true. When the midwife arrived, children would start crawling out from holes and corners of the houses, barns, and other outbuildings. Sooner or later their father would appear, smiling happily like I'd done him a big personal favor. The mother and I would start the conversation. The children stood around smiling shyly, they'd giggle and the small ones would tug at the larger ones' dresses. After you visited for a while, you were a member of the family.

I remember when Richie and I went over to visit Rebecca and Reuben just a few hours after baby

Benjamin was born. That was late in the summer—a busy time to have a baby, what with filling silo.

As we walked up to the house, we watched the mounded loads of corn jouncing along to the silo on a flatbed wagon. We watched the three gleaming, thick-limbed horses—their flesh the color of the earth and the earth the color of gold dust. The warm, juicy smell of the cut stalks filtered through the yard.

Another wagon was in the field working the rows. Another team pulled it, and right alongside of it there was a binder—a machine that cuts the corn stalks, lays them down in clumps on a short conveyer belt, binds the clumps with twine, and then dumps the bound clumps into a waiting Amishman's arms. The corn stalks are cut one by one; the teams go about the field in one direction, working in a square, in the dust, patiently going row by row by row. Standing on the back of the wagon, even for an afternoon, you begin to see the land intimately, as if it were the palm of someone's hand—with wrinkles, cavities, and mounds.

The binder, as I said, is pulled alongside the wagon by the horses; its blade is powered by a small gasoline engine. Reuben, who looks more like a rabbi than an Amish farmer, loped back and forth along the back of the flatbed wagon, catching the clumps of corn as they came off the binder at the front end, carrying them to the far end of the wagon, and stacking them there.

Dr. Kaufman had done the delivery that morning while I'd been on another delivery. Well he didn't actually "do" the delivery. This baby, the sixth in the family, a ten-pounder, and the first boy, had things pretty well under control. They said the baby had insisted on cleaning up after himself, but Dr. Kaufman felt he should do something to earn his pay.

When we arrived Rebecca was lying on the couch. She was dressed in her Amish blue dress, the green shades were all pulled way up, the windows were open, and white sheer curtains luffed in the summer air. She seemed slightly subdued, but otherwise no different than the Rebecca who'd been putting up apple sauce two days before, when I'd stopped by.

I'd just picked up the baby when the other children came flocking in, raising a cloud of dust and noise about their father. The oldest girl had taken over the management of the house. She had magnificent dark, intelligent eyes, natural elegance and poise. She looked like she should be the doctor. On the outside—among the English—she would become a doctor or lawyer or college professor, probably the latter. When she was younger, her mother said, she'd sneak off to the barn and read books instead of doing her chores. "She's learned better now," her mother said. "She doesn't do that anymore. Her sister does it and now this one knows what it's like to miss a pair of hands."

Two of the little girls tumbled onto the couch near their mother, boring instinctively toward her lap. She restrained them from a direct attack on her belly, patted them, and talked to them in Pennsylvania Dutch, the language the Amish use in their homes. The remaining toddler, unwilling to make the dart in front of us to get to her mother, glommed onto her father's leg and all but strapped herself to it.

The younger children, having found their respective safe corners, stared at Richie and me with steady concentration. To be sure, they do not see or talk to that many English and we must have seemed very strange to them. Think of the elementary facts—my hair is short, short as Richie's sometimes; I often wear pants; I talk fast; I make faces that Amish women don't make; I drive around in a car. And the toddlers would know, in some dim way, that I (or Richie and I) was associated with this new baby, and they must have been assembling the pieces: new baby, English woman, small case, mother's flattened stomach. Perhaps I had something to do with the baby being a boy. Jesus came in there somewhere too, they knew. Jesus brought babies. Bewildering.

The older children, having had several opportunities in their lives to get the puzzle pieces together, stood quietly with sage little cat smiles on their faces.

Richie spoke up.

"Filling silo, are you?" he said to Reuben.

"Yeh. Picked my day, didn't I?"

"Can I help?" Richie asked.

"Can you drive a team? One of the men has to go off this afternoon."

"With some instruction, I believe I could," and Richie followed Reuben out to the fields.

I had not seen many women like Rebecca yet; I guess there probably aren't many Rebeccas in the world, not in any population. She was a master of her profession, a housewife and mother of perfect grace. Soft-spoken and unprepossessing, she directed this intimate multitude deftly and joyfully. She had simple dignity and invisible but formidable strength.

Would somebody please bring her something to eat? Cornflakes and a sandwich maybe?

It was 1:30 in the afternoon and she'd already done a morning's work, including having a baby, and it was about time she wanted her breakfast and lunch. The two older girls vanished round the corner to prepare the food.

The cornflakes were quite soggy when they arrived and there was purple stuff glopped all over the top of them. This was grape slush—concentrated grape juice. It appears on all manner of incompatible but otherwise fine food in Amish households. I began considering a vow to never watch an Amish woman eat her first meal after a delivery. Stewed placenta is one thing, decomposing cornflakes with grape sauce is another.

The sandwich came out. Peanut butter and jelly, she'd said. I saw the brown layer and the red layer, one for peanut butter, one for jelly. What was that white layer oozing out between the brown and the red? It was a mayonnaise layer.

I turned away, went to the window, and looked out. Richie was standing, legs bent loosely at the knees, at the front end of the flatbed wagon, a mountain of corn listing from side to side as he guided the team down the lane. He tugged the reins and the team went around the corner of the field and toward the silo.

Rebecca, meanwhile, must have realized that the children had gone wrong with the mayonnaise because she soon called for a piece of bologna (our salami). "Don't try to starve me," she said. "I can eat the kitchen clean." I didn't know how she was going to make the correction in the sandwich, but at least she had all the right parts now: peanut butter to go with the jelly; and bologna to go with the mayonnaise.

She stuffed the bologna right into the sandwich, cheek by jowl with the peanut butter and jelly. She was such a grateful person, a woman of such dignity. Why was she doing this to her food?

One of the children asked for a bite. Another one had to show her mother a toy. Ruthie, the second-oldest girl, came to ask where the box of crocheted hot pads were; two or three other questioners came and went. Rebecca spooned food in her mouth as she could.

These women do not get much of a break from their responsibilities. I remember saying loudly to one woman shortly after she had given birth, "Why, you look so good, you could jump right up and get back to your chores."

She looked at me very crossly. "Hush. Don't you let a soul hear you say that. I feel just fine and I intend to enjoy myself lying here; this is the only vacation I get in a year."

Rebecca's cornflakes were mush, I tell you, warm, spongy mush. The woman could endure anything.

I could see Richie jumping off the wagon. He was now unloading the bound clumps of corn stalks and dropping them on a short conveyer belt. The belt carried the stalks forward through a modest opening into a narrow metal chamber, which was fixed with a mouthful of whirring, glistening blades. The blades shredded the corn and stalks and then a blower shot the cut silage right up to the top of the silo. The whole business was powered by a tractor motor, to which a belt was attached.

An Amishman will use a tractor this way, for its power, but not to work his fields or get from one place to another.

Rebecca, who hadn't finished her cornflakes, now asked for a chocolate cupcake. Well deserved. Wise choice, I thought, assuming the woman would politely set the unfinished food aside, letting her children realize the inadequacy of the meal without faulting them in front of an outsider. The oldest daughter brought the cupcake. Rebecca stripped it of its paper cup, broke it in half, and dropped it directly in the cornflake–grape slush swamp.

That appeared to be the ticket, for she energetically cleaned up the contents of the green bowl and began vigorously scraping away at the bottom of her plate—a traditional ending to meals among the Amish. She smiled enthusiastically. I sighed.

I left in a short while, waving at Richie in the fields with the draft horses. Just think, my Richie the airline pilot and three Amishmen bringing in the crops.

When I came to pick him up later he told me that the boy at the next farm over had an accident while he was working with the corn chopper. He was dead.

I thought about how Richie had been feeding the chopper.

"Seems like if the corn gets stuck on the conveyer belt, the only thing to do is to step over onto the belt and jump up and down to loosen things up. Thing is, if you don't jump off in time, or if your foot gets caught among the stalks, then you fall and get sucked right into the opening and your legs get chewed up right with the corn stalks." Richie paused and looked at me. "Doesn't take long to bleed to death when your whole leg's whacked off," he said.

I tried to be matter-of-fact: "How old was the boy?"

"Fourteen or fifteen, I guess. He's the youngest in his family. It was his first year working full time in the fields. There'll be a viewing tomorrow night. I told Reuben I'd be happy to drive them over."

XI ✄

The Viewing

I was over on Stone Mill Road making a house call the day I had my first viewing. I think it must have been soon after I got to Lancaster because it was spring. My patient had just had her first baby girl and thought that she was the most wonderful thing in the world and that I was a close second. I was basking in my destiny.

So I was in this woman's kitchen wiping cookie crumbs off my face and hugging and chatting with the fat baby on my knee, when an Amishwoman knocked abruptly at the door and walked in. Her face said nothing. It had that flat look, the one the women use when they're shopping in Intercourse, the one that means, "Don't come near me."

By this time I understood the function of the look: it's a way of keeping distance. The Amish use it occasionally among their own, that is, with certain private situations; and they use it regularly with the rest of us. They do not wish the world to know their problems or their joys or even their shopping list; they do not elect to concern themselves with the world.

The woman asked me if I were Dr. Penny, which is what some call me. I said I was and she said, "Maybe you'll be stopping over at Sarah Riehl's on your way home?"

Sarah was eight months pregnant with her second child. Every indicator was healthy. I couldn't imagine why she would have anything wrong, but I'd learned by this time not to ask questions in this sort of situation, mainly because I wouldn't have gotten answers.

You see, Amish do not acknowledge one another's pregnancies. No one has told me why; it's "just their way." When I first came, I would say to my women—who keenly loved news of one another's families—"Do you know so-and-so over in Leola? She's got the same due date as you do."

And they would look at me as if not understanding a word and turn away.

Finally one of the older women grabbed me by the ear and took me aside for instruction. "Hush, dear, we won't be needing any talk about who is going to have a baby. You'll have to learn to stay quiet until after the babies are born."

I had a pair of sisters who rode together forty-five minutes in their buggy to Stephen's office for ante-partum checks and forty-five minutes back to their houses together every month. Day came that the first one delivered, I was sitting on the bed, tucking a baby girl into a pink receiving blanket, and I said to the new mother—figuring an exception would be made in this case—that I wondered whether her sister might be having the twin to this one that same day.

I might as well have suggested that we all go out ice skating. "Now what would you mean by that?" she said, and from then on I conformed to their way exactly.

When the Amishwoman came to say wouldn't I be stopping by at Sarah's, I could only assume it had something to do with her pregnancy and that it was an urgent matter. It meant "Sarah's pregnant and she's in trouble. Go now."

I left quickly, nothing spoken, everything understood, and drove to Sarah's. The barnyard was jammed with buggies and more were turning in. Team after team were hauling husbands and wives to somebody's parlor when everyone had fields to plant.

I parked my car in the forest of black buggies and went to the side of the main house. Sarah and her husband, Joel, as is typical for a young couple, didn't have the main house. They were living in the addition, the part that had been added at some time or another for somebody's parents. These "grossdaadi" houses are typical in Amish country. The old people, the grandmas and grandpas, when they retire from farming, move out of the central house—the one that's built for six and seven children and for having church for fifty and weddings for one hundred and fifty—and into an attached apartment. Actually it's a smaller version of the central house. It's got built-in china closets and everything.

Sarah and Joel had one of these smaller versions. It was fully equipped. Besides the shiny linoleum kitchen floor, on which all Amish home life takes place, besides the china closet, the scrubbed countertop and shining sink, the long table for eating on, for cutting out squares for quilts, for shelling beans and folding clothes, for changing babies—besides all this there was, centered on the long wall of the room, Sarah's clock, the one that Joel gave her when she agreed to marry him. (Girls will not say they are engaged, but they will say they got their clock.) Over a small sink in the corner was a mirrored cabinet and below it a rod with a towel hanging from it. The towel—white and elaborately embroidered with green thread—was wrapped in a plastic covering. She would have given it to him as her token when she accepted the clock. Also on the wall there was a lumber store calendar that had a photograph of a stream running through a glen; there was a board with hooks and dowels for guests' hats and cloaks; there was a blue felt painting, which had Joel's name on it and Sarah's and the name and birthdate of their first child. There was plenty of space left underneath the first child's name.

Joel worked at the farm here where they were living and he was learning blacksmithing to make more money so they could get a place of their own. What with all that to do, Joel still always brought Sarah to the office in their buggy. Once they insisted on sneaking me out the back door to show me the buggy; it was lined with green crushed velvet and was equipped with a matching blanket. (Joel the rake, I began to call him, in memorial to his courting days. His hair was red and I could tell he trimmed his spiffy little beard.) He always asked if he could go into the examining room with his wife and he'd lean over the table, inspecting things, pointing out where the baby's elbow or bottom would raise his wife's belly like a mole raises the earth, and generally he asked a hundred questions about what was going on. He wasn't doing it like he was a plant manager, he wasn't checking to be sure I knew what I was doing; he just didn't control his curiosity and enthusiasm.

That's one difference between Amish and city people, especially those who are having home deliveries: the questions they ask. The Amish are reasonable.

I think it's because they're used to the idea of birth and to taking care of things at home. It's a home- and family-centered culture, and the way they have babies is an extension of the way they live. Newborns, for example, live the early months of their lives on the kitchen table—everybody passing by talking to them, squeezing their tummies, picking them up for a bit of carry-around. If the baby's awake, you'll find him at the table for meals, his food stirred right up with the whipped potatoes, his swing sitting there next to the bench, his gurgles mingling idly with the silence and the talk of his brothers and sisters, his mother and father.

In a couple of years, he'll come running into his mother's room within a couple of hours after the new baby is born. Birth is routine: it doesn't happen every day, but it happens often; and it happens in the barnyard, so it's normal and people have an idea of what it's about and they ask a reasonable number of questions.

Joel and Sarah knew about having babies from their own experience, and Joel's curiosity about the whole thing was just that. He thought having a family was terrific.

Sarah was maybe twenty-two. That day when I stopped by I found her standing quietly in her kitchen, her arms folded in front of her the way the women do. She was in black and she was surrounded by men and women dressed all in black. As the women arrived, they shook hands with the others and nodded. I stood there for a little while, pleading internally with somebody, anybody, to please tell me what to do. Finally, somebody came over.

"Joel was building a silo this morning with three other men. They were near done and Joel was up on top when the brickwork collapsed. He fell and was crushed. Must have died right away. We thought maybe you would check to see if Sarah was okay."

Oh, sure. Okay. And I sucked my breath through my teeth.

About that time, the door swung open and in came six Amishmen carrying a wooden casket. Plain wood with a gray stain on it. They slid it onto the kitchen table, opened the lid, and the viewing started up. Believe it or not, I'd never seen a dead person. All that time in hospitals and no corpses. That had been just fine with me. And this wasn't just a dead person. This was Joel.

A couple of Amishmen walked over to the coffin, looked into it, said things like, "Yep, that's Joel. Doesn't look like he felt a thing." And, "I suppose he has some questions saved up he'll be wanting to ask." And then they stepped aside. I forced myself to get in line. What else could I do?

Sarah, seeing that I was quaking and pale, came and took me by the elbow as soon as I got past her husband. It had been Joel, all right, his red beard brushed up.

Sarah gestured for me to follow her.

When we got to the bedroom Sarah said that she wondered if I would check to see if the baby was all right. There was to be a full viewing tonight; hundreds would be coming. She wanted to know if the baby was all right and that it wouldn't hurt it. Calmly she lay down on the bed so I could examine her and listen to the baby's heartbeat. I did that and I asked her the right questions, but I couldn't concentrate. I was staring at the bed.

The Viewing

Not only had Sarah changed into black mourning clothes, not only had she made the house immaculate for the people coming to the viewing, but she had removed the second pillow from her bed.

XII

The Home Delivery

Over the months, I worked out the problems associated with home deliveries.

Take the ten-minute sterile scrub. I was accustomed to scrubbing in the hospital, and in spite of my impatience with it, I knew it was for good reason. One of the major discoveries of modern medicine was that women were dying in childbirth not because of having babies, but because of germs carried by the people helping them have their babies. Since that discovery, we have all scrubbed up to get the bugs out from under our fingernails and skin cells and, thereby, to keep the mother's wounds safe from infection.

Lying awake in those early months, tossing and turning at night, I figured out how to do a homemade sterile scrub. Even though there would be no nurse standing at attendance, I could still scrub for ten minutes at the kitchen sink, leave my hands dry in the air, take my gloves from the sterile packing and slip them on with minimum contamination.

That plan was good except if the baby started coming fast and if I needed something right now, something that lay deep in my medical bag, and something that could not possibly be described to an Amish farmer. Then my sterile scrub was in jeopardy. I tried to be careful, but I felt bad at the idea of having to commit infractions of my rules.

Then I went to a house where they had no running water. Now, here's the problem: I would have had to prime the pump, scrub up, prime the pump again with my elbow to get water for a better lather, scrub some more, and prime the pump again with my elbow, and rinse my hands. And I was supposed to reserve enough strength to deliver a baby.

Not a chance.

I finally talked to a woman who also did backwoods deliveries and asked her, somewhat frantically, I admit, what she did about the sterile scrub.

"Think about it, dear," she said in a kindly way. "Where do the germs in the hospital come from? They don't come from healthy mothers, now, do they? Healthy mothers have their own immunities; they have immunities to their family members and to germs in their homes. Hospital germs do not come from homes and husbands, they come from people who are in the hospital because they are diseased."

Oh, yeah. It dawned on me. Oh, yeah.

She went serenely on: "Pump the water with your hands. Wash up with soap and water. Pump with your hands. Rinse your hands. Put on the sterile gloves before you do a vaginal exam, change them if you have to paw through your bag or go out to the barn, change them more frequently if your mother's got a tear, and stop worrying, dear." She put her hand softly on my arm. "Stop worrying. Women can have babies at home; they've been doing it for centuries."

I saw virtually no postpartum infection among my home delivery patients.

My patients and I also survived emergencies. I had one terribly shy woman; she blushed at the slightest bit of attention. I had arrived when she was going into labor. I did my routine investigation and found the cord coming down before the baby.

Prolapsed umbilical cord. It means that as the baby's head moves down the birth canal, it presses against the cord, which carries life-supporting oxygen. As the baby's head moves even farther down, the pressure increases until the baby gets no oxygen. The mortality rate for a baby with a prolapsed cord is about 50 percent.

I would have to send the Amishman to the phone for the emergency team, put my hand inside the mother's vagina, and push against the baby's head, holding it back from its descent, and hoping to keep it off the cord until somebody could do a c-section.

So I assigned tasks: he was to get things ready to go; I was to keep the head held back; and she was to pray. I told this woman, with all her painful modesty, that I was going to keep my hand in her vagina during the ride to the hospital and to surgery. She looked at me in the eye and, without a blush, said, "Do what is necessary," and I took a breath and inserted my hand into her. Then, to give us some privacy, I had her husband throw blankets over the two of us. I suppose I hoped we'd look like a bundle of laundry when we arrived at the emergency room door. We stayed that way, lumped together, while we got her on a stretcher, into the ambulance, and all the way to the hospital. She continued to have contractions. She never complained; and what's more, she never blushed.

I regret to say that when we arrived at the emergency room door, a brisk wind snatched away the blankets and left this poor woman and me peculiarly and nakedly attached, in the middle of a parking lot beneath the light of an illuminating moon.

I moaned.

She looked at me directly, as if to say, "Don't you dare start up now." What she actually said was "Don't give it a thought."

Fifteen minutes later she had a baby girl by cesarean section. I had held that baby back by continuous pushing for forty minutes—up to the moment they put her on the delivery table—and it wasn't until she was safely delivered that I remembered I'd been nursing a wrenched shoulder. I remember it vividly because that, probably more than anything, reassured me. Apparently, these things had been arranged so that strength would be there—both in my patients and in myself—when we needed it.

Eventually I noticed that my home delivery statistics were spectacular. I hardly did episiotomies. At first, I thought it was a fluke—that I'd had a run of women with Olympic-class birthing bodies. In those first months of doing home deliveries, Stephen and I nudged one another black and blue as we watched women, eight centimeters dilated (the baby drops out at ten centimeters), bending and bustling, stoking up the stove, making the bed, and stepping into the bathroom for a quick shower. We were used to English women, eight centimeters dilated, who believed they needed help to sip juice.

But the run kept on and I started looking at my

Apgars. An Apgar is a rating scale that measures the condition of a newborn. You consider the baby's heart rate, respiratory effort, muscle tone, reflex irritability, and color, and you give the baby a number between one and ten. Remember all those flat babies in the hospital? The ones that had to be suctioned, bagged, and jiggled about? They averaged Apgars of five or six; my home birth babies: eight or nine.

I carried oxygen to bag the babies. I carried a DeLee's suction to clean out their air passages. I could do episiotomies. I could stitch up tears or cuts. I could give shots for pain. I could get emergency help when I needed it. I was just about positive that I could do anything for these women that a class-one hospital could do—not a big-town, city hospital—but a class-one hospital like Country Hospital. It was getting to be a decided possibility that I could do it better.

I had a friend at one of the bigger hospitals in Philly who arranged for me to conduct an experiment. I thought if I could see a city hospital delivery now, as an anonymous observer, with nothing to do but think, record, and evaluate, I would better understand my growing preference for these Amish home deliveries. Were they—as they seemed to be—better for the mother and baby? Or was I just infatuated with the gentle people?

My friend made it possible for me to watch a delivery. I was not to do anything; just watch.

At City Hospital, I entered a vast room, brazenly white, with fluorescent panels overhead. Waxed floors, empty of humans, stretched away in the distance into disappearing arteries of linoleum. A floor buffer whirred in one of the corridors. Two or three women in white dresses and white caps were posed behind the massive, curving, chest-high desk that centered the room. Their heads turned in one uniform movement, their eyes followed me as I shuffled awkwardly toward the elevator.

I felt like a spy.

The maternity ward looked considerably friendlier. Bright yellow walls and rust-colored carpeting took the hospital edge off the hallways; a waiting room, fitted with a fish tank and trees, was relaxing.

I went to the lockers and changed into a pair of anonymous blue scrub pants and V-necked shirt. I'd get a hat and slippers, as would the father, before we went into the delivery room.

"She's at seven," the duty nurse told me, as we walked back to the woman's room, "but when they ruptured her membranes, the water was green, very green, very meconium, you know. I'm surprised they're willing to have an observer with that kind of a problem."

Meconium-stained fluid meant that the baby had had a bowel movement while in the uterus and it could also indicate fetal distress. In my experience, however, if the heartbeat was good, real alarm was inappropriate. Many fine, healthy babies were delivered with meconium-stained fluid. Alertness, yes; alarm, no. In the hospital, meconium staining meant automatic intervention.

As we approached the room, I could hear the hollow pounding of a baby's heart—it sounded as if it were beating inside an empty refrigerator. The fetal heart monitor, a metal box standing on four metal legs, stood directly to our right as we walked into the room. It was attached to the infant by way of red and green wires that ran along the mound of the mother's stomach and disappeared into the birth canal.

The nurse turned first to the machine and, picking up the long strip of paper that issued from it, examined the graphed lines that ran its length. Absently she asked the mother how she was doing, absently she acknowledged the small sigh and a humble "Okay," and then, finally, having satisfied herself with the paper, she turned her attention to us. She introduced me, smiled at the father, and said something about things being just fine. He looked at me, winked to let me know that he had everything under control in here, and resumed watching the basketball game. For a moment, his wife tried to find me with her eyes, but gave up. The nurse adjusted the band, about two inches in width, that went the girth of the mother's belly. This belly band is another device to measure and record contractions. Like some of the other tracking tools, it inhibits the mother's movement and therefore tends to slow labor. The nurse patted the woman on the arm.

"The doctor will be here shortly," she said, and then left.

The night before I went to City Hospital, I'd delivered Susie and Ephraim Glick's baby. Susie had a bunch of things yet to do before she had her fourth baby, and she was especially determined to get into a quick bath. She had her husband running here and there, looking for some plastic bottles to put hot water in—Susie had varicose veins and we would need to put some heat on them after the delivery. I asked her if she felt like pushing yet and she said no, she didn't, and besides she needed to have a bath. She'd been working in the strawberry patch right up until I'd arrived and her feet were dirty.

I'd set out my things in the bedroom, and sat down

to read a magazine article about growing tomatoes in a raised bed. Susie's husband, Ephraim, marched placidly up and down the stairs with a flashlight, bringing down plastic bottles. He moved the eighteen-month-old out of the bedroom and brought in some things I needed, and just before he sat down, Susie called from the bathtub, "Ask Penny if she wants any tea, Ephraim." I didn't, so he sat down to read the *Botschaft*, the weekly newspaper that serves Old Order Amish communities. There wasn't a sound in the house except for the ticking of Susie's Seth Thomas clock. Occasionally, in the distance, we heard the rumble of thunder. A storm coming our way. That went on for about twenty minutes.

She came out scrubbed from being in the bath and damp from being about ready to push.

"Come on, Ephraim," she said. "Let's go have this baby."

At City Hospital, the woman in the belly band looked slightly confused, then turned to her husband. "Am I having a contraction?" she asked.

He leaned over her and looked at the machine. "Why, yes, you are, dear. Now then, let's push."

One thing you had to say for the father, he had cared enough to memorize the natural childbirth book backward and forward. "Breathe," he said, eyes on the monitor, "that's good, now push, now breathe again, now push." He was so well prepared with book learning that after this child, his perfect son, was born, he would refer to his wee arms and legs as "extremities." "The extremities are normal, dear. Now I am counting the fingers and toes: one, two, three four..." He'd read that this verification of fingers and toes promoted bonding between mother and child.

The mother wants to know if her baby has everything it's supposed to have; his intention was to produce this information for her. He didn't attempt to touch the baby himself; he did not address it directly, nor praise it aloud; instead he assessed it.

I don't imagine he was an unloving man; but what I've seen time and again is that the technology of the hospital overwhelms patients' natural instincts; they are intimidated, afraid of appearing stupid or clumsy or sentimental in a surrounding that seems so efficient and immaculate and intelligent.

His wife screwed up her face and grunted.

She didn't feel the contractions. Because of the regional anesthetic she'd had, the only way she could tell that her body was proceeding with its labor was by the machine. Her urge to push was so numbed that she had to fake it—"Just imagine you're making your bowels move, dear," the nurses would say.

A couple of times during her labor her husband told her, "It's a contraction, dear. Now, then, let's breathe, push, that's good." And then a nurse or other official would come in the room and say forget it. She stopped instantly and resumed her fuzzy stare into space. Her husband pecked her on the forehead and lifted his eyes back up to the television.

Susie and Ephraim's bedroom was too warm, and Ephraim went about and opened a couple of the windows just an inch or two. Great drops of rain began to fall to the earth outside the window, the wind gusted, the white dotted-swiss curtains billowed at the window, and the smell of wet earth filled the bedroom. There are always deliveries—count on it—on nights with thunder and lightning. Something about the barometric pressure. We got Susie settled in her bed, arranged her pillows, and her husband lit a bedside lamp. For the next contraction, I rested my hand on Susie's belly; when it was past, I would do a vaginal exam. For a while, I massaged her feet and legs; her husband dusted his hands with talcum and rubbed his palms into the small of her back.

When Susie's contractions got more serious and closer together, I moved right next to her, one arm resting on my knee; the other, now gloved hand resting on Susie's knee. "Push into your bottom, Susie," I said. "That's good. Now breathe. I can see the baby's head now. I can see your baby's head coming."

The doctor arrived at City Hospital. Tall and artfully graying, he eased in, put one foot on the bed rail and stared at the screen on the monitor. He didn't touch the woman. "Let's get her into the delivery room," he said pleasantly, walking out.

The delivery room walls were dark green shiny tiles with white grouting. The floor, an intaglio, was shiny black with gray and white pebbles floating in it. Shields of stainless steel hung on the far wall; some were punctured by electric receptors, others had metal clips that held stainless-steel instruments, some had ropes of rubbery black cord hanging from them, black cords that swooped down on the floor and coiled loosely around the base of flat-faced lamps that surrounded the delivery table. It, too, was of stainless steel. It seemed so narrow, like a camp cot, and a thin mattress exaggerated the impression. Metal stirrups —which had the shape of molded leg guards—rode the air.

The woman was lifted from a rolling bed onto the delivery table. The doctor, nurses, and onlookers slipped on caps, slippers, gowns, and masks. The attending nurse became a doughy clump of blue. The husband took the shape of a blue monolith near his wife's head.

The woman's body, drugged and heavy, was rolled awkwardly onto the delivery table. Her legs were sunk into huge canvas socks that tied at the knees, and then they were lifted into the leg stirrups and bound with belts and buckles, twice on the foot and twice on the thigh. Once she felt a push breaking through the anesthesia, and then she was asked to pant her way through it so that they could get her bound up. The nurse spread a drape over each leg and then the doctor stepped forward and cast the last drape over her body. It covered her to the neck. From his view, there was nothing of the woman to be seen except for a small area of pale, jellylike flesh with two dark hearts—the vagina and the anus. The great lamps in the room flashed on.

The woman was secured in the lithotomy position. Someday in the future this position will be cited as an example of how our civilization got its technological cart before its medical horse. The lithotomy position —convenient for medical intervention in childbirth— works against the physics and physiology of childbirth. In it a woman can seldom push effectively. She hasn't got any leverage, she hasn't got gravity on her side, she's not in a position to help her pelvic bones spread out, and what's more, the baby's head is pressing for the entire ride on one of the largest blood vessels in her body—thus slowing down circulation when the baby needs it most.

Because she cannot use gravity, because her labor is tempered by immobility, because she hasn't had anything to eat and her blood sugar is low, because she can't let her body follow its unique musculoskeletal formula, because she has assumed that she is not delivering this child but that the doctor and hospital are doing it for her—for all these reasons, her body does not labor as well as it might. And then, of course, the need for surgical intervention increases.

Susie knew her stuff. She rolled over on her side for a while, then onto her back. When the contractions came, I just stood back. Energy rippled the surface of her skin, her arms and legs pounded against the mattress with the leftover pulsations. "Okay, Susie. Let's get you up on your knees. We need to take some pressure off those veins and also give those bones the best chance to spread for the baby's head." Susie sat with her bottom resting on her heels.

The doctor picked up a syringe. It was five inches long. With his back to the woman, he flashed the point of the needle, squirted some of the fluid in an arc in the air, and then turned, not warning the woman that she would feel a prick and a burn. He reached into her, pulled away the exterior flesh, and twice drove the needle into the flesh of her perineum.

The woman's husband hadn't said anything since we came into the delivery room. The woman, the tip of her nose barely visible above the mountain of drapes, said nothing. The baby's head was crawling persistently out of the birth canal.

The doctor hadn't touched her except to put the needle into her.

Now he picked up a pair of scissors and cut from the birth canal toward the woman's left flank, through five muscle groups and an inch and a half to two inches into her. It was a textbook medio-lateral episiotomy.

* * *

At Susie's, I worked the perineum with my fingers, helping it stretch. The baby, held and squeezed by its mother's muscles, came bounding down the birth canal. It turned, ground under the pubic bone, and then its head began to bulge. The perineum thinned. I put my fingers on the cap of the baby's head to keep it from coming too quickly, to give the perineum a chance to stretch. I asked Susie to pant, which slowed the baby's coming.

Left medio-lateral opens the birth canal up, all right. Flesh hung loosely from the cut. The vagina was wide open and lazy and the baby's head rested like a beached whale on the vaginal tissue and in a dark pool of blood. Fresh blood seeped into the drapes.

"Pant," I told Susie.

"Hoosh, hoosh, hoosh."

The baby's head rotated, showing its slant of forehead, then more and more. The perineum slipped over the brow of the face. "There now, there, Susie, there's your baby's head."

Ephraim couldn't stand it anymore, he had to have a better look. He dropped his wife's hand for a minute and came over to look over my shoulder to see the head.

The doctor stood back and reached at arm's length in the general direction of the baby's head. He slipped his fingers under the baby's chin and pulled it out. "There," he said dramatically, "that's what caused the trouble. This baby was trying to push his arm out in front of his head. He's fine now."

* * *

"One more push for the body," I said.

Susie, not losing any momentum, surged one more time, and the baby was out. It started crying right away.

"It's a girl," I said, putting the baby on the bed next to Susie and covering it with a receiving blanket while I cleaned fluids out of her nose and mouth with a syringe. Susie stayed on her knees, a small amount of blood puddling about her, then—giving its standard warning with a narrow rush of fresh blood—the placenta followed. Susie said little. She had one arm free and, drawing the baby toward her, she cuddled her at her side. Ephraim said, "This will make Grandma's one hundred eighth grandchild—that is, if somebody didn't beat us to it."

The doctor handed the baby to the nurse, who carried him to a small metal table in the corner of the room. A heat lamp went on and the baby kicked slowly; he was uncovered and exposed for the first time in his life. The delivery lights came on. "He's cold," the doctor said. "I'd like to warm him up under the heat lamp." The nurse put a plastic suction tube down the boy's throat, a machine hummed, extracting mucus. Without talking to him, she trimmed his cord, wiped his face, and weighed him. His mother had not seen him yet except at a distance; she hadn't touched him.

The doctor delivered the placenta, settled down on his stool, flashed his needle in the lights, and began stitching. He would stitch muscle for fifteen minutes.

Ephraim cut the cord, we wrapped the baby a little better, and I gave her to him to carry about—"leave her head a little lower than the rest of her body so that she won't choke on any mucus"—while I washed Susie up and placed the bottles with hot water in around her legs. Her muscles were shaking from having used up all her sugar supply, so I covered her up with piles of family quilts and got her some apple juice.

The doctor finished stitching. He pulled his gloves off, walked to the baby, and gripping the boy's chin between his thumb and index fingers, said, "You're quite a boy." He went over to the father, shook his hand, told him he'd examine the baby in the nursery, and stepped out.

The nurse started undraping the woman who was shaking and complaining of being cold. Her husband said, "Yes, dear, you're supposed to be." The nurse said nothing, and continued unbuckling the straps that held the woman in her stirrups and untying the giant canvas socks. Finally, the nurse said, "As soon as I've finished here, we'll let you hold your baby for a minute," and finally, she got a light flannel blanket and put it over the woman's body.

Susie and Ephraim's baby would be called Katie. I washed her up, amusing her with my conversation as I did, weighed her, and then put her back on the bed to check her. Discussing who she resembled, how good her color was, and who the grandparents were, I dressed her and wrapped her in a receiving blanket. I put her under the crook in her mother's arm, and she started nursing.

The nurse left the husband and wife in the center of the now echoing delivery room and took the baby down the hall into the nursery. When I left at 1:30 A.M., the baby was on a metal table under bright lights and heat lamps. A woman in the nursery was measuring him. As she left the delivery room, the nurse had said, "Mother can see baby in the morning after doctor makes rounds."

I left Susie and Ephraim's house after the baby had started nursing at the second breast. "The best thing to do," I said, "to keep the baby warm and to help her get gradually accustomed to the outside world, is for the three of you to sleep together tonight. Don't worry, you won't roll over on her—you'll know she's there."

XIII ❧

Getting Married

Neither Richie nor I liked the idea of getting married. Everybody we knew had already been married and nastily divorced. I couldn't stand others' horror stories, let alone the chance of having one of my own. We both thought the wedding ceremony was ridiculous.

But I wanted to go to a midwifery convention on the West Coast and if we were married I could fly on Richie's pass. And since I had stopped being a student, I didn't have any health insurance, and if we got married I could be on Richie's plan. And then we'd about decided to rent a house together and that would be more convenient if we were married. But I hated the idea of getting married, and so did Richie, and I was busy delivering babies and I didn't care to think about it.

About that time, I delivered my first primigravida at home. A primigravida is a girl who is having her first baby. Lizzie was especially proud of the fact. Just by the way she carried herself, she implied that she expected to be awfully good at having babies. She also gave the impression that she tried just a tad harder than everyone else to be sweet and that she was kind of successful at that, too.

When her labor started, she expected undivided attention and she gave me no peace. Her water broke, shouldn't I come right away? No, not yet. Her contractions were starting, should I come right away? No, not yet. And so on. I finally gave in about 5:00 A.M. and went to her house.

The bedroom was still dark when I came in, but I could see the crib, with its doll-baby smooth sheets. One infant gown was arranged in the center of the mattress; next to it were two diaper pins, closed and clipped together, diapers, and an undershirt with ties. A blanket, banded in green ribbon and embroidered in the red, pink, yellow, white, pastel running thread, was folded to show the words *Our Baby*.

Our mother-to-be was sitting up in bed, hair tucked in a white scarf, pillows plumped nicely around her. She had one hand resting gracefully in her lap and the other in her husband's hand. She looked a great deal as if it were Mother's Day and I was there to serve her shirred eggs and blueberry scones in bed, and then the children would be permitted to come in, give her kisses, and run off to play nicely.

She smiled to assure me she was going to be mature, then she spoke, explaining that she was counting on having her baby by sunrise. The pains had been very hard already and she knew it must be just about time. She tucked her lips in with finality, raised her eyebrows, and looked at me as if to pat my acquiescence into place.

She was so bright, so ready, so sure of herself, that

I knew we were hours, if not days, away from a delivery. I put my hand on her stomach and waited for a couple of contractions. They were miles apart and mild.

"Well, now, Lizzie," I said very seriously. "I'm afraid it's going to be some time longer than that." I had to bite my lip so as not to smile. Not that it's funny, but you see it again and again, and you know what they have ahead of them, what they have to face up to in the next few hours—especially ones like this who are thinking about dolls—and you can't help but smile and shake your head a little.

She took it pretty hard. She looked abject.

"Maybe by noon," I said, nodding encouragement, "maybe by noon."

Her shoulders dropped a trifle, she looked at her husband as if asking him to make me understand, her eyes started to water up, but then she took a big breath, gave her shoulders a shake, and looked back at me as if to say that she was a grown-up who was prepared to take life's major setbacks. She was a good girl, I could see that. She had planned on being brave through the hard parts, and here, she said to herself, it was.

Fortunately, the mite hadn't the faintest idea of what hard was.

I gave her some blue cohosh—an herb that stimulates labor—told her to drink juice, get in the bathtub for relief from back pain and, when she felt like it, get out and start walking around the house. The labor was slow; something was keeping it from picking up, and the odds were it was because she knew—for all her bully front—that she was just a child and children can't be mothers.

Lizzie needed time to grapple with herself. I went and got some breakfast.

When I got back, the pain had begun its inevitable education. The rigidity in her shoulders was eroding, and pride was washing out of her face. For a while, she sat slumped in a chair to make a mild show of her suffering, and then, getting no satisfaction from me, she rose and started walking timidly about the room. I told her, "What a good idea," and she perked up, walked with more conviction. When a contraction would start, she'd find her husband's face with her eyes, then go over to where he was sitting in an arm-chair, squat next to him, and put her head in his lap. Time after time, he cradled her head in his lap and with his hand he rubbed the small of her back.

Sometimes, she would look up at him, imploring him, just as the pain started up. Her lip would tremble. The boy would say softly, "There now, there now, you're doing so well." Then he would look at me for reassurance and I would nod.

He turned to me. "She always wanted babies. Ever since I knew her, she wanted babies. It was all I ever heard—babies, babies, babies—way before we were married." She smiled modestly and this time when the contraction came, she stopped next to him and curled up into a self-contained ball. She put one fist on her knee, rested her forehead on it and let the contraction boil out of her body. He watched her, try-ing to stifle the look of pain that crossed his own face as he heard her moan. He waited for her contraction to subside and he stroked her shoulder once, tenta-tively, reverently.

He believed in her. He believed she knew about babies. He believed her big talk. She was his wife. He loved her and couldn't see at all that she was taking new and sorry measure of herself.

She doubted herself. As if the physical pain wasn't enough. She knew she was not being magnificent, transcendent, which was what she had planned. She wondered if maybe she wouldn't even be able to push it out the way any ordinary girl would.

Neither of them had had the slightest idea it was going to be like this.

I sat with them and waited.

There's at least one time before the final appearance of the baby when inexperienced mothers decide for the first time in their lives to give themselves up. They are tired, they have been brave, they've used themselves up, and cry out, "I can't. I just can't. Make it stop. Help me." When the young women say it, I celebrate inside. Because then, if only for a split second, they capitulate to the independence of their bodies and the awesomeness of this business they are joining in.

The ones who are new at having babies, the ones who had darling figures like this one, adoring parents, and special attention—especially them—they war with their bodies, they keep control. Because they are young and strong and willful, because their fathers adored them, because the boys used to flirt with them, these young girls believe they are clever mistresses of their destiny like no mistresses before them, and they try to run the labor with their minds, with their schoolbook ethics of how brave women behave. And then, as the labor proceeds, their strength ebbs and they have to give up. For a while they despise themselves for having failed, and then, finally, they know it is beyond them. They abandon themselves to the force that has overtaken them. They give up their special place in the universe, surrender themselves to those who are helping them, and see themselves in a truer light—they are no more and no less than any struggling woman in labor. The secure ones feel release and throw themselves with grace and abandon into the current that so far outpulls them; the more frightened ones resist the power; they flail and hold themselves back.

Lizzie had been resisting. Trying to be brave and trying to look good when having a baby. As she gave way, her labor progressed. She'd let her shoulders go, her mouth was now unpursed, her legs fell randomly on the bed when the contractions were over.

She was tired. She'd been at it nearly twelve hours. A searing contraction came, and, finally, she cried out, "Help. Help me. I can't do it anymore. Make it stop. I can't go on anymore. Penny, help me." She looked with terror in her eyes to her husband, gripped his shirt, and pleaded with him. He looked at me. "Hold on to Ervin," I said. "Hold tight and, yes, we can do it, you are doing it, your body is guiding you, your baby is coming. Follow your body, put yourself into your pain, bury yourself in the pain. Listen to me: the more you push, the sooner you can put your baby in your arms." I looked at her husband.

"Come on, Lizzie, come on," he said. "Our baby's almost here. It's our baby coming, Lizzie, our baby's coming."

She had her baby about twelve-thirty, a nice baby. Later Ervin helped me out to the car with my suitcase. I looked out my rearview mirror as I drove off. He skipped the pathway and jumped up over the three steps to the front porch. Coming toward me down the lane was a buggy carrying a woman. It would be Lizzie's mother. I'll never figure out how they know when to come.

Lizzie and Ervin had their people. When Lizzie shattered the first time because she couldn't quiet her baby, when she became frantic when a high temperature hit, when she first felt that anguishing suspicion that the baby was changing things between her and Ervin, then she could look to her parents' lives and to her people for help—people who dressed the same way she did; people who performed the same chores in the same order in a day and in a life; people who prayed the same prayers and applied the same rules, people echoing into the past and into the future, showing the way in an endless succession of mirrors.

Black buggies file unevenly across the soft-webbed November morning. Grass and roadside weeds lay down heavy with the weight of the early winter damp air. Small square windows of the buggy frame a husband in his black frock coat and black, flat-brimmed hat. He's been up since four to get the milking done and his face is soft and at rest. His wife, black bonnet in a dark halo around her face, is by his side. She pulls her shawl snugly around her.

In November and December in Lancaster County, on Tuesdays and Thursdays and taking all day, the young people marry. By eight the yard fills up with buggies, and husbands and wives climb out for the wedding ceremony. They enter, the women shaking hands and nodding in fellowship. The marriage sermon goes on for most of the morning—men and women listening on benches on different sides of the room—and, plying verses from the Bible, it is instructive of marriage duties.

Bride and groom, dressed in new but otherwise ordinary Amish clothes, listen—I imagine—the best
they can. Through their excitement, they will hear
some of the obligations recited to them. They needn't
worry too much; what they'll miss at their own wedding, they'll hear at another's. Since it is the custom
in the community to honor the teachings of the
church, the instructions will be used again and
again.

Their minds, I'm sure, concentrate as best they
can on the promises, but as much as anything else, it
is the singing voices of their brothers and sisters,
voices like shuttles working open and shut, each voice
crossing over the bride and groom again and again,
that probably weaves them into being married.

At the bride's house, supper for 100 or 150 is
nearly ready. Family and neighbors have been killing
chickens, chopping celery, cutting up cabbage, scrubbing potatoes, building tables, and setting up tempo-
rary wash stations for days. Now, young men, some
of them dressed rakishly in white shirts and black
string ties, pose casually in the bride's yard or lean
against the side of the barn. They're conscious of the
young women—sequestered upstairs in the bride's
house—watching them, and so they exaggerate their
ease. In a bit, they'll choose a partner whose hand
they'll hold while walking in to the wedding supper.

More guests come. The women carry in desserts
and treats from their kitchens. Cookies, candied popcorn, taffy, and cakes—cakes trimmed to look like
pandas, cakes ringed with flowers made of icing, high
cakes, low cakes, flat cakes, mounded cakes. Shoofly
pie and more shoofly pie. The women, modestly getting one another's name and road and cousin or aunt
until a family connection is rooted out, file along the

display of sweets and admire the kitchen work of others.

Bride and groom, holding hands, go to their corner, called the "Eck," for the wedding dinner. Long tables, covered with blue-and-white checked oilcloth, stretch away from them in either direction, and through the other rooms of the house. Celery stalks, standing straight up in clumps, are the center of the tables, marking the distance off. A hundred or more water glasses are lined up; silverware, napkins, salt and pepper shakers, containers of apple sauce fill the tables. This will be the first sitting.

At the married people's table, men sit on one side, women on the other. They chatter and gossip, men as well as women, until the sound dies down. Somewhere in the room a head drops and instantly all 100 heads drop in silence.

The silence is thrilling. Whatever one's belief or lack of it, the silent prayer before and after each Amish meal does feel holy. It may be that silent prayer is generous to the stranger; it invites him in.

Suddenly, the meal is in full swing. Women and men scoop up their slaw and mashed potatoes—no time for talking now—beets, bread and butter, stuffing, donuts, celery in egg and vinegar cream sauce (a wedding special), coffee and cream, eating as if eating were a hoedown. Servers—more cousins and aunts and uncles of the bride—carry bowls and trays to the table, shovel food on empty patches of plates, and chide those who don't eat enough.

Somewhere in the room there is the sound of one plate being scraped; then the sound of all plates being scraped. Then that one invisible head drops. All heads drop and there is silence again.

Within minutes the tables are cleared and the

dishes, silverware, cups, glasses, serving dishes, spoons are splashing through a washtub in the corner of the room.

In a while, after a second sitting, men will pick up the benches and line them up, and for the afternoon, men and women sing. The voices thicken and dry and begin to sound like wood grain, if wood grain could sing. The men wander in and out of the house—talking in the yard, talking in the barn. They smile and laugh above their beards. The women talk about laundry and babies, gardens, and other weddings this fall. They nurse their babies in the corners, carry one another's cranky baby on a walk. It goes on this way; they will have supper together, too, and there will be more singing.

Late in the evening the young people go to the barn and play games, dancing games with no instruments; they flirt and pair off, getting going for another round of marriages.

The bride and groom spend their wedding night at her home and they spend the next couple of months of weekends visiting family and friends to make themselves known to the brotherhood as a married pair. Then they will set up household.

Lizzie, my child-mother, could marry in trust and begin to take her place in the adult world even though she was not ready. I, Penelope Bradbury—worldly, independent, and self-sufficient modern woman—could not.

Where I came from, the idea of belonging, of carrying and being carried by others, had been sacrificed or lost. No, it was worse than lost, it was considered bad. To trust others, to follow an instruction, to ask for help with the burden of one's life, was to show oneself a fool. It showed you didn't know your way around.

Each of us pretended that we could manage life's events—births, deaths, sickness, and transcendent joy—on the strength of our personalities. Like that girl pretending—with her face all ironed and posed— that she was going to have a baby by sunrise.

Richie and I, if we married, would have to be married by ourselves, alone; if we faltered, we would have only our own peculiar strengths to guide us; and if, between the two of us, they didn't happen to be the right strengths or if they didn't happen to be enough and if we gave ourselves up to others in a moment of trial, as Lizzie had to Ervin and me, others would bear no responsibility for us. We realized that we would be taking our risks alone and the trouble was —although we never talked about it—both of us valued a lasting marriage so much that we truly didn't want to take the chance of having one and losing it.

One morning about ten-thirty I got back from a delivery and Richie was standing in my living room in his blue jeans, a faded L. L. Bean chamois shirt, and a pair of sneakers. He was holding the phone book in his hand. "Justice Douglas K. Wenger of Paradise— metropolis of the farmlands of Pennsylvania, home of one stoplight, one gas station, an ice cream parlor, and the Paradise Hotel with country music every other Saturday night—Justice Douglas K. Wenger has agreed to marry us in half an hour, so if you'd like to change..."

Richie's often a joker in moments of anxiety.

Not talking, I changed from one set of dungarees to another, put on my BMW T-shirt, my L. L. Bean chamois shirt, went out, got in the car, slammed the door shut, and looked straight ahead.

Richie tried to make jokes as we drove along and I tried to be pleasant. Not that I didn't love him; I just detested this.

Judge Wenger, seeing that I was tense and that Richie was trying to make light of things, got into the spirit and said he sure hoped we didn't want a lot of talking at this wedding because he had just been fixing to go fishing when we'd called.

We finished in about ten minutes, paid our fifteen dollars, and took time to go the extra miles and take a honeymoon drive through Intercourse. Then my beeper went off and Richie had a flight to make anyway, so we went our separate ways.

We told hardly anyone that we were married for a year's time. We did tell Richie's mother and father. They had done the same thing back in Island Falls thirty-five years earlier because she had been a nurse and they would have fired her if they knew she was married. After another year, when we felt we had a little record of success behind us, we gradually told others.

XIV 🙘

China

After we got married Richie and I rented a house over on Cowpers Road. We looked landed because we were surrounded by other people's cornfields, but all we had was a small triangle of lawn and a garden plot not much bigger than the back of a farmer's hand.

Did I care that it was small? It had been five years since I'd had a garden and I thought every dirt clod was a diamond. I went out in broad daylight—fearless of the teasing likely to come from my neighbors—my shovel on my shoulder. I turned over the dirt and, over the months, turned in orange rinds, coffee grounds, and lettuce leaves. I planted tomatoes, peas, corn, lettuce, onions, and potatoes. Late in the spring our new neighbor, Eli, came to the door with four seedling tobacco plants in hand; a tribute, I liked to think, to my courageous pretense of having a garden. He planted them for me.

It would make a good joke for the summer weeks, about how Dr. Penny was a tobacco farmer. I'd put my hands in my pockets, lean back against Stephen's waiting room wall, and talk tobacco with the Amish-men coming into the office with their pregnant wives. "It wonders me," I would say, shaking my head thoughtfully, "how our tobacco is going to take this wet (or dry, windy, sunny) weather."

"Why"—they'd pause and think about it some—"do you have tobacco already?" And new respect would fill their eyes.

"Why, yes, we do," I'd say and smile, benign and peaceful as the Buddha.

I stretched my work in the garden. In the morning before breakfast I wandered out to see in what new leaves the dew had gathered. In the afternoon I weeded, I dug, I pulled off imperfect leaves, I watered and sprinkled and cut sharp edges to the garden with my spade. I put up poles for beans, tied up string, and waited for the curling pale green shoots to make openwork against the Amish landscape and sky.

I worked and dug and thought. In the garden, nobody asked me questions, no one challenged me, no one demanded, no one second-guessed. In the garden I had my own mind.

In the garden I had to make the decision about how I was going to practice. I couldn't put it off much longer: the doctors at the hospital still resented me; they chipped away at Stephen every chance they could get and, naturally, that created tension between us. If we were going to continue to practice together, we'd have to put a lot of energy into a new strategy. Did I want to do that? I'd been trying to figure it out. How should I deliver babies? I couldn't choose for others, but I could choose for me. What was right? I'd done my comparative study at City Hospital. I'd read everything I could about births in other cultures: I knew about Native American baby having, imperial

Russia baby having, old white South and old black South baby having, not to mention the baby having of Glasgow wifies and central Philly teens.

The fact was, it had been relatively easy to walk out of that hospital in the city and be glib about how the machinery of medicine was overpowering good sense and mother nature. It was easy to be seduced by the homemade-bread atmosphere of an Amish household. But leaving the practice with Stephen, leaving the hospital altogether, meant turning away from everything.

When I got down to it, there on my hands and knees among the radishes and carrot shoots, I found myself thinking about my women friends, my sisters-in-law, my cousins—all of whom went or would go to hospitals for their babies. I was trained in hospitals. Hospitals saved lives in miraculous ways. I wanted hospitals, English hospitals, to learn to treat my friends and relatives with gentleness and to treat their laboring bodies with respect. I wanted lifesaving technology nearby for them if they needed it. I didn't want to give up on helping get the two styles together, I didn't want to walk away. It didn't seem such an unattainable dream.

In trying to figure out my dilemma, I'd gone so far as to write to a woman who had been a missionary midwife in China before the revolution and who was planning a return tour. China, I thought, might give me some answers—there, I understood, they combined traditional and high-tech medicine; they might know the blend we needed. Maybe we could do what they do in China. If Anna Stone, ex-midwife to the Chinese, would take me with her, I'd pay the $3,000 and find the time to go. I needed answers badly.

I waited to hear from her. Meanwhile, working

along in my dirt, my backside pushing up against my neighbor's rows of new corn, I would experiment with thinking about the problem of modern medicine and baby having the way an Amishman would think about it. It was a question of technology, after all, and the Amish were experts in choosing technology.

Most people on the outside—the English, that is —believe that the Amish culture stays the same. It appears that if you're farming with horses, if you're driving around in a horse and buggy, if you're wearing long skirts, that you're living exactly the same life that your forebears were living in Switzerland in the sixteenth century when they first became religious purists.

The Amish do change. They use different standards than the English to decide how to change, how much to change, and in which direction. But they change.

For myself, I couldn't figure out the bathrooms. Why would Amish people refuse to have electricity brought into their homes by wire, do without phones in their homes, and yet have completely modern bathrooms? I tried making up my own explanations, but none of them made sense. So finally I asked, "How come all of you have nicer bathrooms than I do?" It's because of the government, they said. The government said if they wanted to sell milk from the Amish cow to the English world, it wouldn't do to have outhouses. The Pennsylvania Amish decided they needed milk for a cash product so that husbands and fathers could stay home on the farm, and so, after long discussions and prayer among themselves and final ruminations and prayers by their bishops, the Amishmen installed spiffy new bathrooms in their homes.

131

For another example, in Lancaster County they use generator-run milking machines and cooling tanks—but they don't allow the use of pipes to get the milk from the cow to the cooler; instead the milk is transported in buckets by the children.

We outsiders aren't very good at reasoning through to these decisions in an Amish way. Some of them— like this one with pipes and buckets—seem capricious. When I try to follow the train of thought, make it work in my English logic, I often lose my way. Then it helps to remember a typical Amish explanation for some decisions. "It's just our way," they'll say, as if it would be absurd for us humans to pretend that we understood all the reasons for our ways.

It also helps to remember that the brotherhood is conservative; they've found a good way to live and want to preserve it. As a result, there's a strong tendency to stick with the way things have been because that's the way things have been. I heard one Amishman criticize some of the others for worshipping the past—as unholy a worship, he said, as the worship of any other false god.

Most Amishmen, though, keep their heads turned away from the world and its innovations. It is the few, those irrepressibly curious and innovative by nature, who scan the rest of society to find ways to preserve the Amish life. These experiments show, perhaps better than anyone, how an Amishman makes decisions about technology and change.

I know an Amishman who has a generator-run computer in his chicken coop. He, a quiet, thoughtful, hobbit-sized fellow, agrees with many worldly writers that the computer—the cold, wired, electric-faced, non-organic computer—might be able to help a man stay at home and be with his family and with his community. He is testing his idea, without noise, without announcement. He just keeps his computer in his chicken coop and is teaching himself to understand its possible uses. He has thought most kindly about us non-Amish and hopes that the computer might help us stay home and be with our families, too.

Most of all an Amishman wants to protect his faith, keep his family close, keep his ways, keep humble before God, be a steward of the land, and make a living. If he needs a technology to allow him to continue, then maybe, he'll say, taking a long time to decide—debating the matter with his brethren— maybe he'll use it; but if it gets in the way of faith, family, and stewardship, then he'll stop thinking about it.

About the time I was putting in the first lettuce in my garden, they brought in a new chief of ob-gyn at Country Hospital. He was, as they say, a "take-charge guy," and he thought the thing to do was to make some ruling on every delivery where there was any sort of complication. He made his ruling only after jamming his fingers into the vagina of a laboring woman, needed or not.

Haseena, a sixteen-year-old translucent-skinned girl from India who dressed in a rippling stream-water blue sari, had just come to this country with her American husband. She knew virtually no English. Her husband found me to deliver their baby because in India men do not deliver babies. It is immoral, immodest, and shocking to a woman if a man attends her at birth.

I was very gentle with this soft, murmuring Indian child. I wanted her to feel safe and welcome in her new country; I wanted to lift her, carry her, ease her graciously into being an American and into motherhood. Through her husband, she asked me for books about having her baby. I looked, but could not get hold of books written in Hindi, so I gave her books in English and her husband translated them and read them to her. With great pride, he complained about her, "She keeps me up all night, reading and rereading the books. She is so amazed and hungry to know. Again and again she says, 'Is that the way it is? Read it to me again.'"

I found Haseena waiting at the hospital, at term, in labor and as calm, polished, and beautiful as a cherrywood lily drifting in the late summer sun. She was so still, I thought her labor had just begun. Her calmness soothed me, and I thought that clearly all was going to go well. When I examined her, though, I found that she was almost completely dilated and I also found that the baby was breech.

I pulled the sheet back over her, told the two of them what I'd found, and quietly we began to prepare ourselves.

I knew how to deliver breech babies vaginally. What's more, I was a *woman* who knew how to deliver breech babies. I knew to keep my hands off the breech. I knew how to let the baby's legs and body drop and hang, suspending its weight; I knew to allow the baby's head to notch out, nape hair by nape hair, from under the mother's pubic bone. For myself, I knew how to concentrate on watching the articulation of childbirth in reverse; to keep the ultimate discipline, that is, to observe while physics and mechanics, uninterrupted, synchronized the birth.

If the patient is ready, if the patient trusts, and if I could keep my hands off, it could go well. If it became necessary to surgically intervene, there was time, but there was time for the breech delivery, too, and that would have given us the possibility of leaving this smooth young girl intact and uncut.

The chief arrived. Without speaking and without apologizing for the intrusion, he pulled back the sheets, spread Haseena's legs apart, and rammed his fingers into her. "Breech!" he called out, as if he were yelling at a hockey game. "Primigravida breech! Prepare for c-section." He dropped the sheet, turned, and walked out of the room.

I watched them drop their scalpel into that doeskinned girl, and all the time they were at her, I thought how an Amishman would have seen the situation; he would have known that it is wrong to use technology when it isn't necessary and especially where it violates stewardship.

I did go to China that summer. By the time I left, I suppose I had convinced myself that China would resolve my dilemma once and for all. I fully believed that in China the chasm between natural, traditional health care and modern medical technology did not exist. I must have begun to think of all China, its one billion people, its one-third of the globe, as a thriving Lancaster County taken one step farther. In this China of my mind, the practice of obstetrics was unimaginably rich in technique and wise in application.

Somehow in China, I imagined, they had figured out how to combine—gracefully and humanely—the past with the present.

Anna Stone, the certified nurse-midwife, had served with the American Friends Service Committee Ambulance Corps before the cultural revolution in China. For this, her return trip, she had recruited not only midwives, but old colleagues, people who had been medical service missionaries—including some who had accompanied the people while they fled from the siege of nationalist troops led by Chiang Kai-shek. Some of these Americans had carried X-ray machines on their backs the length of the Long March. In the days when China was ulcerous with crime, warfare, brutality, and disease, Anna Stone and her colleagues were its healers. In China, they were thought of as being Western friends of the highest sort; they were heroes and heroines of China's "darkest hour." The Chinese would respect them and answer questions.

For three weeks we traveled through China by train. At each stop my companions were honored. Special signs went up; banners unfurled. We were treated to formal teas and were honored guests at multicourse banquets; my friends were applauded and bowed to.

At every stop we explained the purpose of the trip. We did not want to see the Great Wall, we did not want to visit the Friendship stores, and we did not want to see showcase hospitals. We wanted to see the miracle of modern China, how everyday health care and medical practice in China had scooped the Chinese people out of a scabrous, infested past and, combining traditional and modern techniques, had made life in China healthy. I, of course, hungered to see how China practiced obstetrical medicine in a way that preserved wholeness.

Stubbornly they kept us away from the people's China. Relentlessly, they took us to city hospitals equipped with labor beds that were hard and metal and were furnished with straps and stirrups. They showed us hospital layouts that made it clear that the father had no place in the delivery room.

I had anticipated learning about the application of herbal therapies in the hospital setting; instead I answered questions about the dosage of magnesium sulfate for preeclamptic patients. I expected to discuss how hospitals planned for patients to walk about and bathe during labor, to see labor beds that permitted delivery postures I had never dreamed of; instead I answered questions about techniques for inducing labor, about genetic research, about amniocentesis, about ultra-sound, about every space-age, silicone-chip obstetrical device. Our hosts spoke without apology of high rates of cesarean section and high forceps delivery.

I was deeply disappointed. I had come around the world to find sanity and wisdom, and what I found was a people elbowing their way toward a medical technology I had already seen, one I too often had found brutal, stupid, and mean.

I suppose the Chinese bureaucrats will remember it as an official gaffe, but one day our group did stop in a commonplace farm commune—the kind of spot we had been begging to visit. We pulled up to a mud-walled, whitewashed, dirt-floored clinic where no Westerner had been before. With the others, I stopped and peered in the door. A padded cradle stood against the wall, rough-cut wood shelves held jars of herbs, and over in the corner of the room, casting a shadow on the chalky walls, was a pressure cooker—exactly the same pressure cooker that I used at home to sterilize my instruments. Next to it, instrument packs, packed in muslin, folded just the way I fold mine.

Curious children came skipping in from a nearby

schoolhouse; they poked and prodded one another as they made their way to the clinic to make a circle around the strangers. I repeated one of the few words I knew in Chinese. "Midwife," I said, pointing to myself. "Midwife," I repeated. "Midwife, midwife," until finally one of the older children ran to the fields.

In a while a woman came bouncing up the road from the fields on her fat-wheeled bike. I smiled, beckoned, and walked toward the door of the hut. She followed me. I pointed to the pressure cooker and to me and nodded; she took my hand. I pointed to myself. "Midwife," I said in Chinese. I pointed to the instrument packs and to me and nodded; she patted my hand and nodded back. Again and again, we patted one another and nodded.

I didn't bother to think. I didn't compare her practice with mine or try to remember what I might transport to the United States. I was overwhelmed. I knew without question, I knew it from the bottom side of my stomach, I knew it with my head and my heart, "This is good. This is right. This is the way." Back in the United States, back in Lancaster County, back home among the Amish, apparently, I had been slowly finding my way through the distraction of high technology and politics, toward the center of the business. I was slowly rediscovering the universal, the truest methods of delivering babies.

XV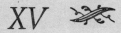

Losses

I got back from China just in time to watch my neighbors start dropping the corn out in front of my house. It had been a generous summer. The stalks were heavy, and when the wind hurried through them, it sounded as if the leaves, in unself-conscious enthusiasm, were applauding their own performance. Richie—now on his second silo-filling season—managed a team of mules casually, with the same loose joints, the same grace he had in the cockpit.

I didn't help with filling silo, but I did throw myself into tobacco spearing. Actually, I didn't have a choice. About a week after I got back, in the evening, just about sunset, I went out to visit my garden. I looked down and realized that my entire tobacco crop—that is, all four plants of it—had been harvested for me; cut and speared while I'd been off on a delivery. The crime or favor—I didn't know which—was still fresh; the leaves were just beginning to wilt.

I was standing there, shaking my head and wondering if there was such a thing as tobacco bandits, when Eli drove up in his farm wagon. Eli pulled on his beard a few times, studied the horizon with great care, and then, apparently fully convinced it was true, observed that it was a fair evening.

I agreed.

He took a little while and then he asked, "Any new babies?"

Well, yes, there had been, as a matter of fact. "An English girl," I said. "Someone you're not likely to know."

He rested and let the answer sink in.

He adjusted the reins, rested, and then said, "See you got your tobacco about put away."

"Why, yes, Eli," I said, walking over to tug at a spot on the horse's harness, "it appears that I do." I looked him in the eye, then back at the horse, and then I waited. I stroked the horse's neck, ran my hand along his back, and patted him lightly on the flank. "I don't suppose you'd know how this tobacco got down, now would you?" I asked.

He smiled just a trifle, looking awfully pleased with himself for a man who was supposed to be concerned with humility. "I just believe I might," he said.

He adjusted the way he was sitting in the buggy, made some remark about how it was a terrible good year for tobacco and especially right here in this particular hollow, said he thought he ought to be going, and he turned his wagon in the drive.

After he'd turned his horse to leave, he looked around over his shoulder and he mentioned they'd be spearing the next evening over to his house if I would still be wondering how it got done.

So I helped put away Eli's tobacco crop.

Tobacco is a major cash crop for the Amish, a significant source of income for the families and for the entire community. If you're part of the community, you share in tobacco growing.

The cycle starts in November, as soon as the kitchen garden is picked clean of the last remaining beets. A farmer then leads a couple of mules into the backyard and gets them to drag disks through the earth. Using giant steam plates he sterilizes the plot, patch by patch, and then tucks it under black plastic sheeting. He literally puts the ground to rest for the winter months. In the spring, with a watering can, he sprinkles seeds over the plot and in June the family members carry the seedlings, which look a lot like heads of butter lettuce, out to the fields in cardboard boxes and nest them, by hand, one by one, in the dirt. From planting to stripping, each tobacco plant is tended by hand.

Over the summer months the beds are hoed, cultivated and weeded; then, in late August or early September, once they have achieved their full size — by now, they look like giant versions of romaine lettuce — harvesting begins; that is, the tobacco is "put away." The men lead the process; they go out with long-handled shears and they cut the fat stalks of the plants that are ready for harvest. (Transplanting is staged so that all of the rows don't come to maturity at the same time.) These lie flat, shriveling slowly in the sun until the women and the children arrive in the late afternoon or after supper.

I'd head over to Eli's in my blue jeans after finishing up office hours or house calls. Along with the other women, I'd pick up a lathe — a flat-sided stick about five feet long — and, slipping a metal tip over one end, I'd make a spear. I worked along the rows, picking up cut plants, spearing their stalks, and pulling the stalks down onto the lathe.

Mary, Eli's six-year-old, gave me a hand. Mary's not much bigger than a squirrel, but she was out in the fields dragging the plants to the grown-ups. If one of my plants got stuck on a lathe, she'd hang on it and swing like it was a gymnast's bar until it fell down. She'd look up at me, giggle, and scurry off to find another stalk.

We the spearers left the lathes on the ground behind us as we worked. Once we finished, Eli and his son would appear with the wagon and they'd walk up and down the rows, lifting the lathes off the ground and piling them on the wagon. They'd go from the field to the drying barn for hanging. There the leaves drape, gradually changing over the months from a moist fleshy green to a golden brown. In the winter months—November, December, and January—families, and young people especially, get their big stove going in the stripping room in their barn. They sing, tell stories, and strip the tobacco leaves; then they press, bale and ready the leaves for market.

It was during the harvesting of tobacco and the filling of silo, I remember, when Reuben and Rebecca came to Dr. Kaufman's office with baby Benjamin on their lap. I was about to rush over and start to babble. I thought I might favor them with a dramatic rendition of how Richie was plying the corn-cutting trade he'd learned at Reuben's side a year before, but I stopped myself. Something was wrong.

Benjamin's weight was terrible; there were hollow shadows around his eyes; his forehead seemed large and heavy, and worse, his awareness would blur and he'd drift away off, leaving us behind. I couldn't believe it. Baby Benjamin, baby boy after all those girls, a child whose arrival had been celebrated by so many light hearts, a baby like this was meant to be snooping through the kitchen cupboards or smacking his fat palm in a bowl of mushy cornflakes and grape slush; he was meant to be crawling all over his sisters, giving them hugs, and yanking on their skirts. He had perfect, loving, generous parents; he came from a household robust with vitality and health. A mistake for this baby to be sick. Reuben and Rebecca sat calmly, answering questions, and we all agreed that the baby should be taken to Infants & Childrens Hospital for a complete battery of tests. I agreed to drive them up the next day.

Unfortunately, I wasn't able to make the first trip. The evening of the day I saw Baby Benjamin, while I was out spearing tobacco, I got fierce cramps and it was all I could do to get home and curl up in a knot on my bed. I didn't even have the strength to fix the hot water bottle. I lay in my bed moaning while great boulders of pain rolled back and forth over my abdomen.

I stayed there in torment for several hours before I finally realized what was happening. I was having a miscarriage. It took me the longest time to figure it out—had I been a patient of mine, I might have been quicker—but the fact is, my reproductive system gives little information from which to diagnose. It appears to be totally random. Some of the world's finest doctors said it "defied description"; others said that if I ever conceived it would be a miracle, and that if such a miracle occurred, the resulting embryo could be expected to last about thirty minutes. By the time I'd put all the pieces together, I figured out that I'd been pregnant for about three months and this was a miscarriage.

Once it hit me, I felt an overwhelming sense of awe. Richie and I had made this little fellow who didn't pay any attention to prognoses of fancy East Coast physicians. Here he was, meant to live for no more than thirty minutes altogether, and instead, he had survived to be an old man, relatively speaking, an irascible old ten-weeker who must have fought death tooth and nail, as far as I could tell from the wrenching, dragging, stamping, and storming that was going on inside me. How I admired him (I knew it was a boy). I rolled over, sputtering partly with the joy at the thought of the life that had landed inside of me and, at the same time, stuffing one pillow hard against my stomach and jamming my face into another pillow, as if that would smother the pain.

I used to say to my patients that miscarriage—that far along—was often said to be more painful than normal labor. I say it with greater conviction now.

When Richie came home from his trip that day, he got the hot water bottle and the talcum powder, and hour after hour, he patiently massaged my back and kept my head tucked safely in his lap. Sometimes Richie can love me so that I become nothing but the warmth and safety of his arms.

We lost our baby together.

I know, you could say I never really had a baby, except during those few hours when it was already over and done with, but I guess these things aren't entirely logical. I loved my baby. Writhing on my bed, yes, absorbed in pain and self-pity, yes, still I was flooded with adoration for this tiny, not yet shaped baby who had lived in me. I was awed by him; awed by the spirit of the child who had lived so long where no child was meant to live. To have had such an amazing being alive within oneself is a great honor; to have been a vessel, a carrying basket—even for a while. Oh, God, I wanted him to have lived. I wanted to see him, wrap him, carry him, study his face. I wanted to raise him, protect him; I wanted for Richie and me to teach him what we had learned about living. I would have respected this child. Oh, God, I didn't want him to be dead. I didn't believe he could be dead.

But he was and we named him. Together Richie and I buried him.

I rested a day. Richie worked around the house and brought me Chinese food for dinner, and then there was nothing to do but go back to work.

When I got back to the office I found they hadn't completed the tests on baby Benjamin. I drove him and Reuben and Rebecca back up to Infants & Childrens. Baby Benjamin looked worse than he had two days before and now I was truly angry with him, angry because he threatened to abandon the earth, leave it, even though he'd been given such a ruddy start. He'd had a good chance for a full, strong life and he appeared to be letting it slip lazily away from him. I couldn't bear it.

I don't know what we talked about driving up to the hospital. The tobacco crop, I suppose. Corn crop. The other children. I don't know.

At Infants & Childrens they found that Benjamin had an invasive brain tumor—one, that is, that had grown into the vital parts of the brain and that made removal virtually impossible.

At the news, the faces of Reuben and Rebecca rippled and stilled. Without saying anything, without touching each other, just exchanging looks acknowledging that each had heard, they rose and followed the doctor where he bid them go to sign some papers.

I stayed with Benjamin. He began to wail thinly

when they left, and I picked him up and held him so he could lay his head against my shoulder and at the same time look out the window on voluptuous green slopes and an autumn forest. I swayed back and forth, lightly stroking his back, and soon the thin wail died out.

I studied his ear and eye, his frail, translucent cheeks. With great care, I touched the soft hair on his head and patted his bundled body; I put my cheek against his sweet warm skin. Finally, I understood that there was nothing I could do for him, and because of that I succumbed to him as he was. I saw his exquisite beauty, I felt the perfection of his terribly imperfect body. He gave me great peace, little Benjamin did, because I could love him exactly as he was, exactly for the amount of time he had with us. For a short while, I was able to love him not for what he might have been, not for what he would give to all of us and become, but for what he was. I could love him for the moment, completely; I didn't have to measure love out so it would last. It seemed to me that the grandest thing I could ever do with my life was to treat Benjamin kindly while he lived; to try to give him all goodness and love while he was here. Nothing more.

Reuben and Rebecca took Benjamin home as soon as they could because he cried himself hoarse when he was in the hospital. They took him home because, although the doctors could operate, there was virtually no hope of it making any difference. When they left, one of the nurses said, "I admire your decision."

But the next day, Reuben and Rebecca started hearing from Baltimore doctors. It was a rare case, they said; perhaps they could find a way to help some other child in years to come if they could treat Benjamin. They asked Reuben and Rebecca to hand over the child.

At home, all the family took turns carrying and rocking Benjamin, who suffered horribly through the days and nights. They, too, wanted to give him as much love as there was time for.

Soon the doctors began to say they could prolong his life for five years, and then, with suspicious quickness, they said they could cure him.

Reuben and Rebecca prayed, talked with each other, the minister, and the children, and decided that the baby had enough to endure without being put in the hands of strangers in a hospital where the family could only visit him. They said they didn't believe that God had given them Benjamin to be used in an experiment.

The doctors filed suit. "They planned," Rebecca said, "to come take him out of our arms. We didn't know about this law. We didn't know they could carry our baby away without our saying, 'Go ahead, take our baby from his family.'"

The rest of the machinations aren't important. I know I ended up driving Rebecca, Reuben, and Benjamin to Infants & Children's, where Benjamin died.

It was after that that I decided to leave Stephen and the Country Hospital. Up until then I'd limited my disagreement with hospitals and doctors to birthing issues; and each time they shocked me with their technological bluster, I reminded myself that if I really wanted change I had to stay and act on what I believed.

But this was one too many interventions. They should not have intruded into the delicate sanctuary of Benjamin's family. There was defilement in that act. And then my feelings compounded, and I remembered how they had rent Haseena's body and raided the tranquility which had been so gracefully carried in her. I remembered how commonly they went to a laboring woman's bedside to read the printouts from the fetal heart monitor and never even looked her in the face or stroked her hair. I thought of all the times they had put their rapacious need to accumulate medical knowledge before their respect for the people they were caring for.

In their great enterprise, too many of the doctors seemed to have forgotten that other people's ways could be worthy and deserving of honor.

I left Stephen and I left Country Hospital. I would go out on my own. I didn't know if any women would come and ask for my care. I just knew I wanted to take care of Amish women and their babies in a way that respected them.

XVI ❧

The Office

We got the last of the tobacco put away about the same time that I decided to go out on my own, so it seemed right to promise everyone an open house and tobacco harvest party on the Sunday night before a Monday opening. I shouldn't say it seemed right; in fact, the whole idea made me very nervous.

After all, Richie and I had only to paint the entire downstairs of the house, furnish it, and talk to insurance, accounting, and legal people. We had to put ads in all the newspapers for used examining tables and lights and other equipment. That left making sure that every pregnant woman in Lancaster County knew that I was thinking—make that thinking *and* dreaming—about her pregnancy, her backache, her other children, her husband, and her baby, and letting her know that I was willing to go to enormous lengths to give her sensitive care and the birth that she wanted.

I established a custom birth policy and, as it turned out, it gave me some of my best births.

Take the bus, for example. Martha Ann, a holdout from the hippie generation, was an earth mother of the sixties sort. She was a vegetarian, she wore beads, she made major decisions based on astrological forecasts; she was mellow, forgiving, and loving. She had children from different phases of her life and that was okay.

When it was time for her last child, she chose to have it at home in her bus on the hillside in the woods of Pennsylvania. She came to me because most doctors don't deliver babies in buses.

She also wanted her last child to be Sunday's child so, late on a Saturday evening, she fixed herself a "California cocktail," which is the whole-earth version of Pitocin. At one o'clock on Sunday morning, then, she called me and I drove out to her place. It was one of those nights so startling in their beauty that I thank God I have a job that gets me up to see them. Stars pierced the sky. The moon lounged lush and full on the horizon. The fields rippled broadly under the night sky; they opened wide and spilled out on a down slope of the planet. I drove out beyond the trees, beyond the intersections, into the open field lands. The road meandered as if it had all the time and space in the world to get to where it was going. A stream shimmered beside me as I drove through the night, and then I crossed a narrow stone bridge and turned onto a gravel lane leading up to the woods.

At the top of the hill in a small meadow surrounded by trees, was the old bus, settled knee deep in wildflowers. My headlights shone across its front and across the meadow, where they illuminated a tepee.

Pulling aside a drape of gauze and wool, I entered the bus. Inside there was a kitchen counter, sink and stove, a table, and a master bedroom—that is, a wall-to-wall bed at the rear of the bus. The steering wheel and driver's seat were in their regular place at the front.

Martha Ann's husband, Chuck, had attached a shed roof to the bus lengthwise and set in walls and a concrete floor. This addition to the home was filled with tables and couches, which seemed to be pushed here and there depending on day and time or on mood or necessity. A child lay sleeping on a couch; another snored lightly from a hammock not far away. The room was toasty, heated by a stove. Moonlight poured in.

A huge jar of catnip tea sat on the counter in the kitchen, where I settled my things. Wood shelves sagged under sacks of oranges, barley, other grains, and dried cereals. A three-year-old blond dumpling of a child named Foxglove crawled up on the countertop, composed herself Indian-style, and confidently asked for more tea and honey, please, Gretchen. Her friend, Gretchen, came from the tepee.

I had checked Martha Ann already. She decided to stay on the bed—accustomed as she was to going quickly once she'd started her labor. I let her alone for a while while I got acquainted with Gretchen—my most likely candidate for assistant. While we talked, Chuck awoke, growled contentedly, stretched his great bear self, and went for his clothes. He put on a pair of Elmer Fudds and a fiesta "birthing" shirt, hand-embroidered with tropical red and orange flowers by Martha Ann.

Gretchen had a grand, quiet smile and dark straight hair; she was a handsome, soft-spoken woman. I couldn't quite figure out how to ask her whether she knew anything about baby having because I couldn't tell how old she was. She looked like she was in her early twenties, but she had a silent, assured way, as if she knew a great deal more than twenty years teaches. She patiently made tea and picked things up, put them away, and wiped the countertop. I kept trying to gauge her age and experience. I didn't want to insult her, but if she was unfamiliar with childbirth, I wanted to prepare her. I had no choice but to be direct. I asked her what she knew.

"Oh, well, what I learned from having five children myself. The oldest is eighteen and the youngest is fifteen months. I had the first two in the hospital and I realized what I was missing." That was all. No political comment. No railing at the medical establishment. She just realized what she was missing and started having her babies at home. She must have been at least thirty-four and she looked no older than twenty-two. I had no idea how she could have stayed so unharassed five children later, but I thought she would be able to help if I needed it.

The final character was Chuck's mother; an oxford-cloth, middle-class woman with streaked hair and button earrings. Carrying a great tureen of soup, she stepped into the bus as graciously and comfortably as if she were arriving at her lawyer son's suburban split-level; she appeared content, proud, and as if all she ever wanted was for her grandchildren to be born in buses. Foxglove got down off the counter, toddled over, and climbed up on her grandma's lap.

Hearing changes in Martha Ann's breathing, I went in to be with her. Gretchen, who had agreed to get another of my cases from the car, was just leaving the bus when the lights flickered and went out. "Under the front seat," I called out to her, "is a flashlight that might work."

Chuck's mother lit the only candle in the place. I pointedly assured Martha Ann and Chuck, now sitting cross-legged on the bed beside his wife, that most of delivering a baby was a matter of handwork rather than eyework, so even if we had to do it completely in the dark, it would be all right.

Gretchen had just beamed the flashlight on the newcomer's point of arrival when swoosh, the baby's head came zooming out of the birth canal like it was on a greased sluice. The top of the baby's head was covered with green meconium stain. Baby-alert.

But the baby's face rose quickly and with good color. I reached automatically to feel for the cord at the neck; it was wrapped twice tightly—a "noosling" we call it, because as the baby moves down the birth canal, the tighter the cord becomes. I picked up one clamp, slipped it under the cord and fastened it. I picked up the other clamp, but there was so little elbow room and so little light that I was afraid of clamping Martha Ann instead of the cord. Tentatively, I put on the second clamp. Then I cut the cord between the clamps, setting the baby free.

Her body slid out quickly. I grabbed her, sucked the mucus from her mouth, throat, and nose, and started to rub her back vigorously to get a good cry. At the same time, I noticed that the far end of the umbilical cord was vigorously spurting blood all over the walls of the bus; it thrashed around like an unattended hose going full bore. Apparently my tentative second clamp had not fully closed off the cord. Blood shot up the wall, across the front of Chuck's shirt, and spattered across my arm. I watched it, wondering how I was going to snare the thing, when Gretchen calmly reached over, took hold of the cord, and pressed it tight between her fingers. She said nothing. The baby cried, I clamped the cord a second time and went back to my routine.

Apparently all events were easily absorbed in this household—straight grandmas and errant umbilical cords—so it was an easy thing to settle the new baby, to give Grandma her chance to admire, to mop the blood off the walls, and to get Martha Ann started nursing. Chuck climbed over his wife and the new baby, giving each of them a hug as he went, and then he wandered on out to see if he could find out why the power had failed. Foxglove, who had finished her tea and honey by now, replaced him on the bed. As she sat, tentatively stroking the baby's head, we women—Foxglove included—talked names. Then Gretchen drifted toward the front of the bus; Grandma—who had to be up at six to get to a special church service—bustled off with her face shining. I gave my instructions, gave Martha Ann congratulations, and went to the shed part of the bus, where Chuck and Gretchen were.

The lights were still out. The moonlight, riding high above the pine trees, cast a shadow work of windowpanes on the concrete floor. Chuck, burly and composed, his arms folded comfortably across hs chest, stood in front of the stove and watched his older children sleep. Gretchen was sitting a ways away, stroking the head of one child. It was still warm in the shed. I stood and watched them until I was absolutely quiet, too, and then I lifted the doorway of gauze and went back into the pure and perfect night.

But this—my night visit to the oneness of things—was yet to come. And if I'd been planning on a clientele of hippies, it would have been different in those weeks before I opened my office. But the

Amish, as far as I could tell, were the reverse of the hippies. Instead of "Everybody come in and do your own thing," it was "Do not taint us with your worldly ways."

No matter how much I wanted to be with the Amish, to protect their women and children at childbirth, to be sensitive to the childbirth standards of their culture, I didn't know whether or not they would fully accept me, either as their midwife or as their neighbor and friend. It wasn't that they hadn't been cordial and pleasant; they had been. But that's something different than real friendship—friendship that would forgive me my mistakes and tolerate me even when I grew short-tempered or tired; friendship that would allow me to drop in unannounced at somebody's house, just to visit or even to ask sensitive questions, like what do you do if somebody won't pay or how do you get a woman to cooperate?

Besides, I wasn't sure about how they would accept me as a midwife on my own. Before they had the assurance of knowing that I worked out of the same office as a doctor. Would they trust me if I told them that I had a back-up doctor—which I had—even though they couldn't see her each time they came in?

Besides, we knew the Amish well enough now—it was about a year after we'd first come to Paradise—to appreciate that their way excludes outsiders.

It might sound as if I was suffering from simple start-up anxieties, which I was, but they were compounded by the basic fact of Amish life: that for four and a half centuries, the Amish had remained separate from the world. I was clearly of the world; I didn't go to church or claim a faith. "Be ye not yoked unequally together with unbelievers," the Amish might quote. And they might continue, "What communion hath light with darkness?" I being darkness and they being light. I had no reason to think that the Amish would compromise their four and a half centuries of separation from worldliness for me.

It's different among the English, who favor new people and new ideas. Even with respect to basic values like family and faith. They've been toyed with, experimented with, tossed about, lionized, examined, measured, bought, sold, and otherwise treated like consumables. One year, it's a great thing for a woman to get married and have babies, and the next year it isn't—at least for trend setters. I stopped trying to follow which religion was current among my friends —Eastern or Western, intellectual or passionate, mystical or pragmatic, challenging or reassuring, embracing or isolating.

Of all the standards that humans might live by, the Amish culled a few staples and succeeded in holding to them—even now, in the midst of a historical time whistling with pressures to change. I watched the Amish, admired them, and finally had to try to understand how they came to have a standard of excellence gained by loving and caring, by unselfishness and humility, by humble and hard work, by commitment to community and to helping one another; whereas the English world has a standard of excellence that requires beating the other guy to the punch.

The Amish way began in the sixteenth century and was part of a much larger reforming tide sweeping through Europe at that time. In the opinion of the reformers, the Catholic church had disfigured the teachings of the simple carpenter of Nazareth and turned the church into a self-serving institution for the rich and powerful.

Martin Luther, in the ninety-five theses he nailed

to the door of the castle church at Wittenberg in 1517, led the challenge. He observed that the spiritual tone of the church had been undercut by such practices as the selling of redemptions from sin. In a later document, he criticized the church's acceptance of the pronouncement by popes that they were divine; he rebelled against the idea that all messages to God should have to go through priests and popes. Luther argued that an ordinary man ought not to have to get past so many earthly brokers in order to pray to God.

To the contrary, Luther claimed, all believers were priests and each man was directly responsible for his communion with God.

In 1523 in Switzerland, Conrad Grebel argued that if it was true that each man was responsible for his relationship with God, then it followed that infants ought not to be baptized because infants couldn't actually choose to follow God. Baptism, Grebel said, ought to be only upon profession of faith, and ought therefore to be only for people who had reached an age of understanding. Those who followed this belief were called Anabaptists.

They refused to baptize their infants and began to follow a simple religious life. They attempted to live as Christ did. Each day, they sought to live in humility, lowliness, obedience, and service. They believed that only those who truly practiced Jesus' teachings of love and nonresistance deserved to be called Christians. They gathered in a brotherhood of believers.

The Roman Catholic establishment loathed the challenge to their leadership and persecuted the Anabaptists. Tortures and executions of the early Anabaptists are recorded in a book of martyrs, still found in every Amish home.

The Amish, who were one of many Anabaptist sects, were notable for emphasizing the importance of being separate from the world. They strictly interpreted standards of social avoidance, or *meidung*. *Meidung* means that if a member of the church falls by the moral wayside, they are to be shunned; that is, members shall not eat with them, nor do business with them, nor converse with them. The standard applies to one's fallen children, one's parents, and one's spouse.

Of course, since I had not been raised Amish, I couldn't fall away and I wouldn't be shunned. But that wasn't the question; my questions were about the depth of their tolerance for my way of life. A people who are so serious about maintaining their status as "strangers" in this world that they are willing to give up relations with their family members are a people who might be unforgiving toward those who had lived a less pure life. So I worried about whether they would be able to come comfortably to my house, have a snack by electric light, and on that inevitable day when I needed them, would they stand by me? For example, if a child was born imperfect and the parents, hurt and angry, attacked me, would the Amish keep coming to me?

"Blessed is the man that walketh not in the counsel of the ungodly."

In the last couple of weeks before the open house and tobacco harvest party, my new English friend Helen came around to help out. Helen, a twenty-seven-year-old nurse practitioner who worked in a local clinic, talked eagerly about going out on her own, so she followed my undertaking with real enthusiasm.

Helen's ingenuous face belied her competence as a nurse. She answered calls any time of the day or night; she measured the medical circumstances with an electronic precision, made decisions, acted swiftly and kindly, asked after the entire family, faultlessly remembering whose hearts, bones, ears, and bowels had last been of bother. She detected problems early on and saved lives, and she made tiresome, repetitive house calls so that her patients could be at home instead of in the hospital.

But in all things except nursing, Helen was as profound as a peppermint stick. She looked most natural when cavorting along the roadside with her puppy.

Patients loved her and she loved them back. Later, when she did go out on her own, she'd chatter endlessly about her visits to a ninety-seven-year-old Amishman. The old man, worker to the last, had been wheeling his crumbling body out to the shed every morning and working all day long on craftwork. It was wear and tear for which his old body had lost its forbearance, and he started getting sick all the time and complained of being dizzy. His family couldn't get him to slow down. Amishmen work.

Helen marched in, all five feet of her, and gave the old man the what-for. She shook her finger at the cadaverous, white-haired, well-respected old man, and said, "Now you're just going to have to take care of yourself. You're not nineteen anymore, are you, old man? Now let's eat ice cream and agree upon how much work you can do every day." She gave him her swell smile and he shaped right up.

Of course, in some things, her Amish patients wouldn't do what she wanted and that bewildered her. She had an elderly woman with a bad heart. The woman was strong enough to have her own apartment in the grossdaadi house, but not so strong that a couple of her grandchildren didn't sleep right upstairs above her for protection. During the day she'd sit at a table by her window, watching the small children play in the barnyard, and she'd snap beans or fold clothes. "Eyes won't do for quilting anymore," she said.

The old woman showed signs of having trouble with her heart and Helen urged her and the rest of the family to get her into the hospital for some tests. The old woman refused. "We can control this," Helen argued with exasperation. "With the proper examinations and medications, we can control this heartbeat and she can live much longer. Now come on."

The old woman smiled and dismissed her. "I believe I'll just leave things to go according to plan," she said, and Helen suffered massive frustration. Helen's imagination just didn't stretch so far as old, contented, and happily accepting of God's will. Neither, for that matter, did mine.

Helen helped me get things together that last couple of weeks before opening day at the office. In the evenings we got out announcements. I finished up some deliveries that I had agreed to do for Stephen. Richie hounded me until I talked to agents about office insurance (I'd long since had midwifery insurance). He painted, scraped, fixed, polished, and scrubbed the entire downstairs office space; he did virtually everything but sew the curtains. Helen and I baked and froze for days, hoping to do the right thing by our Amish guests, if they came.

Everything went just fine. Our magnificent team act worked perfectly. Richie kept things in order, I worked relentlessly, and Helen stayed excited.

Well, maybe not everything went fine. But so what

if all the newspaper ads and telephone calls had failed to turn up used equipment, and so what if that was the case Friday afternoon before the Monday morning that my first patients were to arrive. So what if the only place I had to examine patients on was our waterbed. Actually, they could choose between the waterbed or the waiting room carpet.

So what if I was becoming—in spite of my entrepreneurial pose of confidence—thoroughly uneasy. An Amish neighbor tried to comfort me. She would say, "If it was meant to be, it will be." She wasn't particularly sugary about it, it's just that I could live without insipid comfort, thank you. My Amish neighbor didn't understand in the least. She didn't even guess that where I came from you made things happen, and if they didn't happen right, it was your fault.

Let those who had legions of aunts, uncles, cousins, and grandpas to stand in their kitchen in times of trial sing "What will be, will be," because it was logical when everybody in horse-and-buggy distance was prepared to drop everything and come over to start raising your barn the day after it burned down. (One Friday I was going to make a house call on a woman whose barn had burned down on Tuesday, and was planning on finding the place by using the burned-down barn as a landmark. Wrong. They'd rebuilt it by then.) One could afford the luxury of being philosophical and bending with the wind when everyone in the neighborhood has known you since you were born and when everyone takes a personal and communal interest in your welfare.

I came from the land of the lone tree.

On Saturday morning—forty-eight hours exactly from opening—my Amish neighbor came by. "Call Dr. Ellis's widow. She wants to talk to you."

I did, and the widow said she'd heard that I was going into business for myself and maybe I would like to come over and look at some of the office equipment that her husband had. She'd been meaning to sell it but hadn't and since her husband had been an advocate of midwifery she thought it would be in keeping with his memory if I could make use of some of his equipment.

I furnished my office for $150. What will be, will be.

Which left me only to get through my first attempt at a party for my Amish neighbors.

At the time, Helen didn't know many Amish. "Oh, goody," she said earnestly "a dessert party." Dessert party, oh, dear, no. At dessert parties you serve meringue hearts to women with hollows in their cheeks. The women keep their ankles crossed the whole time.

"This, dear Helen, is not a dessert party; this is a 'snack.' 'Snack,' my dear, means mounding the table high with food." (Our guests, remember, normally do hard physical work twelve to fourteen hours a day.) "Snack for four families means pulling out every flat surface in the house"—I was considering using the newly acquired examining table—"spreading each one with a bed sheet, and when the guests arrive, it means making an endless parade of food to the table. That's 'snack,' Helen."

I tried to remember everything I'd observed about eating in an Amish home so I would get it right.

It poured the night of the party, so Helen and Richard decided to drive out in several laps and pick up our guests. I was limp with anxiety. I figured they all would have forgotten and gone to bed. Joylessly, I waited for the cars to return empty. I tried to think of things to say to Helen and Richard so they wouldn't feel bad. But, no, pretty soon Richard came up the lane and, though I'd become accustomed to the way these people looked by now, I still stood wide-eyed and freshly charmed when I watched Rachel, my first party guest, walk into my living room in her big black bonnet, her black cape with the initials embroidered in the corner, and her baby underneath. Her face was scrubbed.

At first, everyone was very quiet. They took off their bonnets or hats and then took one of the chairs that I'd put in a circle around the room. They sat there without saying too much. "Did you get your examining table?"

"Yes, thanks, I did."

"Good, good."

"Did you get your pump fixed?"

"Yes, I did. Matthew helped me."

"Good, good."

It wasn't like I didn't know about this pace of conversation; it was the way it was always done. But I would have welcomed a sign.

The room soon filled with young women and children and young mothers in blue, brown, and lavender dresses. Old Silla sat down next to old Lizzie in white wicker rocking chairs and they rocked and talked. The girls stood in groups and talked shyly, sounding like birds; the boys stood about with their hands in their pockets, grinning, asking me if I thought I had enough food. Men scooped up small children. Young women bounced them about.

Then, the last carful of people filed in the room. Helen trailed them in, glistening like a candy apple. Helen had been rendered useless. She was in love with an Amish boy. In the time it had taken to drive from his house to ours, Helen had fallen in love with young Sam. And he with her. It was done.

I brought out pumpkin custard, mincemeat pie, Helen's *New York Times Health Food Cookbook* apple crisp, pumpkin pie, Fritos. I brought out chocolate marble cake with chocolate frosting and plain chocolate cake with peanut butter frosting. I brought out pretzels and popcorn. I brought out five gallons of apple cider, and at the last minute, I set out two gallons of Cloister Dairy ice cream, cookies, and pastry bars.

We sat down for a snack.

And then I asked for grace.

When I opened my eyes the beards and bright eyes were still there.

We ate. Bowls and plates filled up, layers of custard plopped flat on layers of pie, which sank into ice cream spooned over cake. Glassfuls of apple juice gurgled up to the lips of tumblers and in some cases overflowed the top, and then everything was passed from hand to hand again and they ate even more. I don't even know what they talked about; I couldn't concentrate for getting everything they needed to eat.

I knew Amish liked games. So, seeing everything was going okay, I got out my balloons and passed them out. "Blow up your balloons," I said. "The person whose balloon lasts the longest wins the game." They looked at me blankly. Surely, I thought, they get the idea. Ohmygosh. Maybe they do not believe in balloons. Maybe Anabaptists had rules about balloons. "That is," I went on, "you want to break the other person's balloon and save your own." I lunged for Richie's balloon.

They got it.

The room went berserk. With flash and gusto, old

men attacked young ones, old women took out after toddlers, teenagers squealed, neighbor fell upon neighbor, husband upon wife, son upon father. They crushed each other, snuck up on each other, slid around, ganged up. Sam and Helen peeped at each other and snuck about in attacks and counterattacks for the duration.

We lined up for Pin the Tail on the Donkey and everyone played, starting with the little ones and working on up. It took the longest time, for the women had to remove their coverings in order to be blindfolded, and then they had to be turned carefully, once, twice, three times. Interest never flagged.

"Oh, that's just the right direction, Johnny, just right. Keep it up and you'll be putting that pin in the side of a real donkey."

"Okay, Reuben, maybe this one time you can keep yourself from going round in circles."

"Eek, eek, Rebecca, you're going to stab me."

Everyone who lived on our road thought Richie must be somebody very significant in the outside world—dressing up in that uniform and flying those big planes through the sky—so they whooped and whooped when he lost his way, nearly stepped on baby Susie, and tried to pin the donkey's tail directly on old Silla's elbow. And Reuben filled a balloon with water and crashed it over my head just as I put my tail in the right place. Sam was there right in time to put his young farmer's hand kindly on Helen's shoulders to turn her around. She blushed the color of strawberry soda pop.

While the adults recovered themselves, the young people wandered about, off into the kitchen and out of sight. We thought they must be getting drinks of water or something, but soon we heard muffled giggling.

Richard and I—having anticipated this very event —looked at each other, melodramatically leaned down in unison to untie our shoes, got up together, and crept down the hall, in step and on tiptoe. Neither he nor I smiled. I beckoned for the others to follow.

Upon reaching the bedroom door, Richie turned abruptly to his Amish platoon and dramatically signaled them to remain silent. We cracked open the bedroom door and he and I took the first peek at a half dozen Amish children, bouncing, rolling about and giggling on the waterbed amongst the bonnets and caps. Richie and I stepped aside and let the others look. Finally, we threw the door open and exposed the little vandals. They squealed appropriately and dove for the four corners of the room.

"Why, what's this?" Reuben said, snatching his boys very seriously from the bed. "Now what would this bed be?" He put his fingers to its surface and tested it.

"Stand with your back to it, Reuben," I said, and he did and I toppled him over. He smiled wondrously. Then he rolled over to one side and back to the other.

"Where's my wife?" he said. "Come here, wife, and see what this is like." She climbed on, giggling like Helen would have giggled, and the two of them lay there smiling foolishly, and then Reuben sighed and said resignedly, "I suppose you'd be needing electricity for a bed like this, now wouldn't you?"

XVII

Mothers and Fathers

They did come to me to deliver their babies. They came to me so many times to deliver their babies that by the end of my first year of private practice I was in need of major recuperation. Five babies the first month, ten the third, increasing up to twenty a month by the time my first vacation came. I drove up to the camp at Pleasant Pond that August, walked into the lake up to my neck and stood there for two weeks, weeping with exhaustion.

It was partly the count. Just the number of hours you have to be awake to deliver twenty babies—for some reason, I won't or can't sleep when I'm out on a delivery, even if nothing's going to happen for a while. Then, in the beginning, I was applying the standards I used when I was working in the hospital; I used to arrive very early and stayed with the patient a long time after the birth so that I could protect them from unnecessary interference in their birth and in their early hours with their child. But those things are only part of it; I was most exhausted by teaching myself how to work well with the woman and her family on her own terrain.

When you go to the hospital to have your baby, they put you in a bed like all other hospital beds, they dress you in a gown like all other hospital gowns, they surround you by an entire hospital staff that guides you along a track that diminishes your individuality and its unique demands, they substitute sophisticated procedures, and relatively speaking, your having a baby is efficient and unemotional for the attendants.

When I started out in practice by myself, I didn't fully appreciate that when I went single-handedly to deliver babies at home—one midwife in the midst of at least three generations of a family—that I would be, in many respects, at their mercy. The qualities of their lives and relationships crowded in on the relatively simple act of birth, making it rich with possibilities—some beneficial, some not.

For, in spite of how uniform the Amish appear to be, in spite of their rigorous discipline over their community's behavior, not all Amish people are the same. Conventional wisdom says that no people are all the same; but when you see people who look like each other and are all quiet and say a lot of the same things when they do talk . . . it's hard to believe otherwise.

In Intercourse, at the People's Place, they have a slide show that helps tourists get some of the Amish facts straight. I usually take my guests there first, partly because I never tire of the show and partly because it explains things so well.

From the show my friends have quickly grasped the idea that food is not religion, although it is an important—and loved— part of Amish life. Fairly quickly, they grasp the idea that the Amish prefer their way of life to the mainstream; they do not envy life in the cities nor do they envy "progress." What is hardest for my friends to grasp is that Amish people are not all the same. They are not pressed, as the slide show says, "out of one Amish cookie cutter."

They are lively gentle people, pious gentle people, funny one, boring ones, mean ones, kind ones, intelligent ones, ones not so smart.

Take intelligent, for example.

I was still working with Stephen when Amos and Barbara King started having trouble with their fourth baby. They'd lost their third baby in the hospital one or two weeks after birth, and now the fourth was having trouble breathing and wasn't eating well. Stephen figured it was a virus but sent it to the hospital for some tests. Amos insisted it wasn't a virus. The pattern, he repeated, was the same as with the child before.

Amos was right; it wasn't a virus. The baby's metabolic system wasn't working right, and though Country Hospital couldn't determine exactly why it was dysfunctional, Stephen had narrowed it down enough so that the researchers he called at Infants & Childrens were ready with specific tests when the baby arrived. Thirty-six hours later, amino acid analyzer tests showed that the mother's milk was killing the fourth child, just as it probably had killed the third.

Amos King—simple Amish farmer, chicken breeder, corn picker, manure shoveler, father today of five children, two of whom are normal and three of whom have the metabolic disorder—has become an expert in this exquisitely complex and changeable condition. So educated have we all become, due to Amos's way, that in spite of the possibility of handicap in their last baby, I felt completely safe in delivering it at home. At the crucial twelfth hour after birth, exactly, a local medical technician, a young man who knew the family and who was, therefore, willing to get up before dawn to make the test, appeared at the Kings' farmhouse door, took a blood sample from the new baby, drove it to Infants & Childrens, and in a record thirty hours after birth we found out the baby had the metabolic disorder and the special diet was begun.

Amos King found the sensitivity I had often missed in the medical system. In his gentle, self-effacing style, he succeeded at what the rest of us have often failed at: getting the specialists to adapt to an unusual circumstance. Amos King does have joy in his face and he is innocent of personal competition or self-serving motives. That's why, I guess, the hospital set aside its normal regulations and allowed Amos King to walk right alongside that second sick baby's blood as it made its way through the labyrinth of usually proud, protective, and intensely competitive researchers. He asked them about the physiology of the disease—although he wouldn't have called it that in the beginning—and explained that he needed to understand because he lived on a farm a long way from Infants & Childrens and he would be needing to make as many routine tests on the baby as was possible for him to do at home, and he would be needing to figure how to adjust the baby's diet accordingly. Researchers, who don't customarily share their discoveries with each other until after publication, got chatty about the ins and outs of metabolic research with this Amish farmer.

Today Amos King probably knows more about certain metabolic disorders than most researchers in the country. He makes intricate calculations for each of the afflicted children as to what they can eat, when, and in what quantities.

The controls aren't perfect—no one knows how to do that yet—and each time a child's system goes out of balance, some brain damage is done. So in Amos and Barbara's home, a number of the children have difficulty talking and walking. It doesn't make any difference—well, yes, it does. The household seems blessed. The children are generally crawling all over each other, laughing and playing. "We just do what we can each day," Amos says easily and saunters off as if he were a man without a responsibility or a thought in the world.

But I've said that the Amish come in all kinds.

Abysmal November. A resentful dawn is ragging at the eastern sky. The phone rings.

"You gotta come here quick."

"Who is this?"

"You don't know me."

"Do I know your wife?"

"No."

"What's the problem?"

"The wife, she just had a baby about an hour ago and it looks sort of funny, and the afterbirth never came yet. The wife, she still didn't want me to call you, but I didn't know what to do."

"Who's your doctor?"

"The wife didn't want no doctor. You gotta come."

I hated these calls. I had no choice. He'd never call the ambulance and I couldn't leave a woman with an afterbirth still in her an hour after the baby'd come.

"All right, I'll come. You get back to that house as

fast as you can. Make sure that baby is wrapped warm and you stay right next to your wife—don't you dare let her get up."

I drove in a straight line overland through somebody's hay field, pounding my fist in fury on the steering wheel as I went. "It's all right to put your baby's life in danger," I screamed, "and to put your wife's life in danger—she's probably just waiting until I get there to begin to hemorrhage, one hour, for Pete's sake—just because you're too something or other to make sure your wife gets to the doctor. So what if she 'didn't want no doctor.' So what!"

I marched into the kitchen. For an Amish kitchen, it was strangely disordered.

"Where's your wife?"

He looked at me dully and pointed the way.

I could see it now. The first lawsuit brought by an Amishman in four and a half centuries.

I brushed passed the father and went to the bedroom.

Absolutely nothing had been prepared for this baby, I could see that. After if had come, the girl must have simply rolled over and pulled a heap of blankets over herself. She was lying with her face toward the wall, clutching the blankets, her new baby apparently hidden somewhere among them.

"How are you doing, Barbara?" I asked.

She didn't answer.

"Barbara, my name is Penny and I'm the midwife. I've come to see you and your baby. We'll have to deliver your afterbirth, otherwise you might begin to bleed heavily. And then we need to see if you and the baby are all right. It'll go better for both of you if we do this together."

Still she didn't reply. She pulled the blankets farther

up over her face, and even through the mound of them, I could see her spine stiffen.

She stayed that way. She wouldn't talk or look at me. I had to search for the child, who turned out to be fine, and delivered the afterbirth without the hemorrhage I'd expected. Apparently it had separated well enough, but she may have resisted pushing it out. Throughout these operations, she never spoke. With perfect consistency, she kept her head turned away from me, as if I were loathsome. She submitted to my taking the baby away to wash it only because her husband made her, and when I brought it back, ready for nursing, she grabbed it to her and turned her back to me again.

Her husband sat in a chair in the kitchen most of the time, his head dropped, his eyes focused on the floor.

Never had I had a delivery like this. It can't happen; even if young people aren't able to get ready for the birth themselves, even if there are mental problems, the girl's mother or a neighbor will step in and get things ready.

"Who's going to help with this baby?" I asked the father.

"She wants to do it herself," he said helplessly.

"She can't do it herself. Surely you can see that now. That baby could have died; your wife could have died. Where's this girl's mother? Who's going to help with this baby? You make it your business to work this out, and in case you think I'm not serious, I want you to know that I'm not leaving this house until I know."

He went into the bedroom and I went out to the car to see if I could find extra boxes of diaper samples. When he came back he said his wife's younger sister would be coming.

I went back the next day. The sister and a neighbor were there. Barbara sat in a rocking chair with its back to the center of the room. The baby was in her lap and she stroked it and cooed. I asked her questions; she answered each of them in a word or two and cooed in the space between answers, successfully making the cooing a battering ram to drive me away.

On the way out, I was able to ask the neighbor how it happened that they were allowed to be so unprepared. "We didn't know them," she said. "They just moved here from another county; we thought their family would be helping them. Now we found out that the girls' mother died not so long ago and we didn't realize how it was with them. But we see how they are and can help." The father was nowhere to be seen.

A few weeks later I went back one more time. The sister was still there and the house had gained some order, but the mother hadn't changed. Again, she talked only to her baby during the visit. It was as if with the soft, beating patter she could keep all of us away, and slowly herself slip inch by inch inside the baby and live within her.

This time I found the father roaming around the back of the barn. While I talked, he looked out toward the fields and ran a leather harness nervously through his fingers. I told him that the baby was doing fine but that I thought his wife would still need some help.

"I suppose you'll be wanting your money now then," he said.

"Yes," I answered, wondering if he'd heard a word

I'd said about his wife. There was little I could do about it. "I'll be sending you a bill and it will be less than I normally would charge because you didn't have the prenatal office visits, but I want you to understand that I should actually charge you more. A woman who hasn't had prenatal care is at much higher risk. Furthermore, I want to make it clear that I will never deliver another child of yours under circumstances like that. Never. Do you understand?"

"Oh," he said, almost blithely. "I don't believe we need to worry about that. Ever since you delivered her baby, my wife never pays me any attention." Then he paused for a moment and his fingers stopped roaming the edge of the harness. He looked at me and only slowly did his eyes move away from mine. His defenses must have abandoned him. His young body sagged and after a while he said in a low voice, "So I believe I'll just be paying you this once."

When I'd be hit by that reflexive fear—"They're gonna get me"—as I was in this case, I'd calm myself by reaching back into the memory of another night that began just as this one had.

Middle of the night, didn't know the man, didn't know the woman. Then: "We had prenatal care from Dr. Blake and he's not here now and my wife and I, we haven't had a baby for seven years and would you please come?"

I went as fast as I possibly could.

When I pulled up in this farmyard, the father's Ichabod Crane body came soaring out the door to give me a hand with my suitcase. When he bent over, his face skin fell in thin, worn folds around his mouth. His sweater, with its baggy pockets and leather buttons, hung as if from a peg off his backbone. Nevertheless, he hoisted the suitcase and swung it off toward the house, leaving, I'm sure, black and blue spots on his legs for weeks.

Once inside, he rushed from drawer to cupboard; he climbed, scurried, put back, folded, unfolded, shook his head in frustration, nibbled, and sniffed; and soon he had something that resembled everything we needed. He stopped now and again when he heard his wife moan and stared painfully and helplessly at her, his long fingers dragging on the hem of his sweater. Then, coming to, he'd wipe the palms of his hands on his pants, and patter off to find something else.

Like the other woman, this one said little. But she didn't turn her head away. "I'm not such a young woman anymore," she said when we began, and then, seeming to fully understand the physiological barriers that age puts up before childbirth, she concentrated on having the baby.

All went well.

As I was leaving, the husband said, "Thank you. We wouldn't have known what to do." And his wife, who had remained silent even in the aftermath of the birth, called me back. "I wanted to thank you," she said. "Every night I'll pray for you and the good work you are doing."

At Booth in Philadelphia, Sue Yates had harped on professional responsibility. Nurses, she said at every opportunity, took orders from doctors. Certified nurse-midwives gave their own orders, made their own decisions; they and they alone had to carry the burden of responsibility for what happened at a delivery. In the hospital, we had to fight for that responsibility because doctors were constantly second-guessing us.

With my home delivery practice, I had unrestricted responsibility—and thrived on it. Among other things, it allowed me to give women what I thought was the best possible care. I wanted responsibility—even when I was so tired that I didn't know if I could carry it anymore.

But I found it peculiarly difficult to know that somebody was praying for me; to have an Amishwoman asking God to look after me and my work. All of these people, all of my patients, believe in God and in prayer, and I don't care what I might have believed—I could have been an avowed atheist when I arrived—when I'm out there among them, it's different. What I believed or didn't believe was beside the point. In my patients' minds, God was in there helping or hindering my work.

It was the final responsibility. That woman said she'd pray for me and these people do what they say they will do. Every night, before she drops into bed she's saying, "And God bless Penny and her work." I try very hard.

XVIII

Giving Yourself Up

Once you understand that Amish people are individuals, just like people in other societies, it's tempting to rush to the conclusion that Amish are like all other Americans. But that's not true either. The Amish are a disarmingly gentle people.

There's a vegetable stand over on Spring Road. I buy there whenever I can—peas in the spring, cantaloupe in summer, cauliflower in the late fall. The girl, Sara, who sells to me must be twenty by now; she mows the lawn and keeps the dirt turned between the Sweet Williams in the beds on the family farm. In the fall, she's out working in galoshes many sizes too big for her, and wearing a dark sweater with holes in the elbows, she rakes the wet, leathery leaves and tends the stand—which is not a lot bigger than a phone shed.

The vegetable stand is my idea of an ashram or a retreat. When the IRS is niggling me, or Richie tells me one too many times not to slam the back door, or when some patient talks back to me or refuses to take her vitamins or asks me to run her errands for her—whenever my insides start clashing about, when the sharp-toothed wheels of anxiety begin whirring, I go buy vegetables at the Spring Road stand.

Sara carefully puts her rake aside when I pull up and walks over next to the stand and waits there for me to say something. She smiles. She's not outgoing, so she doesn't say anything. She just smiles, one arm folded across her waist, the other hanging loosely down her side.

"Hi, Sara. Nice day, isn't it?"

"Hi, Penny. Yes, it is."

"Can you give me one of those cauliflowers today?" I say.

She goes to the back of her stand. Maybe she only has seven cauliflowers to sell altogether. "What size would suit you?" she asks. I hold out my hands to make a bowl for the size I want and she nods and begins to study, one by one, the seven cauliflowers she has to choose from.

Sara is mentally retarded. For her to compare the sizes of cauliflowers and to choose one that is the same size as I showed her with my hands is hard work. She goes deliberately, carefully, and exceedingly slowly. I feel my impatience rising. My mind starts calculating on how little this young woman seems to appreciate my affairs with the IRS, my burdens as a midwife, not to mention keeping Richie happy by going to the movies with him at night when I'd rather be at home wrapped in a blanket. Sara, oblivious to the full scale of my duties or my importance, perhaps even discounting them, continues to study the cauliflowers at her implacable pace.

I don't say anything. Fortunately, I've always been able to stop myself. It's partly because I don't care to behave like a jerk; partly because I came here for the express purpose of getting things in the proper perspective again; partly because I would just bewilder Sara; but mostly because Sara is one of the most contented-looking human beings I've ever seen.

I try to subdue my internal self.

Sara concentrates. I concentrate. Tentatively she picks up one cauliflower, studies it, looks over at my hands in order to remember the size I want, then sets that head down and goes to the next one. Strangely, as she moves intently on, my irritation subsides. The third time—that's when she usually finds just what she was looking for and she knows she's gotten it right—her face is joyful. She holds the cauliflower up like an offering and looks at me expectantly.

It's about then that I come fully around myself. The young woman, patient enough to study cauliflowers, has found the exact size I was looking for. I look at Sara's hopeful face and nod. I can't remember now what I had myself agitated over. I lean back against the side of the stand and start to watch the leaves fall while Sara finds just the right-size bag for my cauliflower and then begins the job of getting my money and making change.

It is the custom of the Amish to "give themselves up" to what life delivers them because if God didn't mean it to be, they assume, it wouldn't have happened. They give themselves up to smaller events. I remember when Sadie Mae's husband was chosen to be minister. Sadie Mae confessed that she was an unlikely minister's wife—did more than her share of running around when she was young; she was the first woman in her neighborhood to start wearing black running shoes with a racing stripe instead of black oxfords. When her husband, Sam, became minister, she had to start wearing old high-buttoned black leather shoes and black stockings to church. "I had a hard time giving myself up to that," she said, pausing, "but I imagine the other women had a harder time. You know, I was never the kind of girl to be a minister's wife. When I was young they had to send a team of people out to drag me back into the services; I wanted to stay outside and talk and joke. And now, you know, that I'm the minister's wife, I'm supposed to lead the women into the services. I believe there's a lot of women in my church who have a hard time with that."

As they give themselves up, they seem to become both more gentle and more joyful.

The bedroom was more mussed than most. Katie had tossed her covering on the broad white windowsill next to a half-filled glass of juice and a Scrabble game. A throw rug, made of tags of brightly colored material and looking like a heap of oversized confetti, was jammed halfway under the bed, a toy tractor and several wooden sheep twisted among its folds.

"Well, now, where would you be wanting to put this suitcase?" said Ike, and he promptly dragged the rocking chair out of the way to make room for my equipment. He disentangled the toys, stuffed them under his arm, straightened the rug, and hurried off to the kitchen for fresh juice. Katie disappeared into the bathroom to change into her gown, calling for a box of tissues as she went, mumbling to me that she would have liked another week before the baby came so she could get her cherries put up, and I clicked my case open, got out my equipment, straightened the bed, shook the pillows, checked my radio, and then all of us regathered at the bed, where it was finally quiet. We weren't going to be waiting too long for the baby, Katie and Ike's fifth.

I just thought I would let her settle, get by a couple more contractions, and then examine her. The three of us sat and waited.

In the corner of the room near the bed was a door frame with a dotted-swiss curtain tied back across its opening. I could see just the headboard and a few bars of a crib showing. As the three of us sat, I heard a gurgling and sputtering from the room behind the curtain. Such a thing is not unusual, often older babies are in the room with us when the new ones are born—sometimes they wake and, seemingly hypnotized, stand holding onto the edge of their crib and absorbedly watch the proceedings. Sometimes when the new baby is all wrapped up, we take it over and show it to the toddler, who will poke tentatively at the arrival.

The child in the crib gurgled again, and I thought, on second hearing, that it wasn't the sound of a toddler.

"Should we get Emma up?" Katie said to Ike. He nodded and without saying anything further went over to the door frame and bent over into the crib.

A farmer's forearms are powerful; his muscles wind down his arm in swirls and band his wrists with strength enough to heft fifty-pound bales of hay off the back of a flatbed farm wagon and toss them ten feet up into the upper corners of the hay barn. Ike lowered one of his forearms into the crib and lifted out a child—not a baby, but a child of eleven or twelve. I stared at her. Her head, square and big, lolled on a neck that had no strength. Then came a frail carapace body. It was followed by long, spindly arms and legs. They jutted and bent across one another as she rose out of the crib; Ike tried to gather them up like sticks of firewood from a forest floor, but one arm and then another would drop and fall as he lifted her out ever so carefully from her crib. He went after them patiently. Her complexion gleamed and her eyes were radiant even in the dark humid night air of the bedroom. Ike's arms—ropy strands of iron by day—seemed to soften into a cushioned basket for the bundle of sticks of the child's body as he gathered and regathered them.

"Well now, Emma," he said, finally having settled her in his arms, and as if returning to the middle of a chat with an old friend. "We believe it's time now." He stood at the foot of the bed so she could see her mother; he patted her back, stroked her arm, and looked at her affectionately. "It's time for the baby," he said to her. And then to me, "We haven't many secrets from Emma." With his great paw, he reached down and pulled a slippery stocking back up her narrow leg.

Then he sat in the rocking chair with her, talking with her and me and Katie. As her mother's contractions began to increase, Emma's face shone more, at least is seemed that way to me. Emma seemed wondrous at what was happening in the room that night. I was stunned by her presence. Honored, I suppose. She was an exaltation. When it came time for the last of the birth, Ike tucked Emma in a chair among pillows so he could help his wife.

The new baby came, squalling and yammering for attention, and as soon as we washed and wrapped him, we took him to Emma and placed him in the nest made by her long arms and legs, held together by her father's arms. Pretty soon the baby fell quiet.

It was nice for Emma too. She would not be having children of her own, of course. She'd been a fine, tumbling child. Then, when she was three or four, she'd been stricken with a raging fever. She was sick for a week, and afterward her parents watched her wither.

Sometime since then they had come to adore her more deeply. Not to compensate, not for the sake of piety. I think she was their special companion. I think their baby was her baby. I think her life, remnant though it seemed at first, filled and joined with theirs and made them all joyful.

XIX

Love

Helen and Sam said they were just friends and fabricated friendlike reasons for being together. Sam, for example, helped Helen train the horse she'd bought at the horse auction. I'd drive by and watch them in the afternoon—Sam with a rope, walking patiently around a corral; she beside him, asking earnest questions about the disposition of sugar cubes to pet horses. He'd explain, I suppose, and she would nod zestfully, as if it were the most intriguing thing in the universe. When their work was done, he'd hitch up his horse and buggy and Helen would perch by his side for the ride home, enraptured; her chin would jut out a little as they drove along and so give her crisp smile a head start; her hands would be folded hard together and sunk deeply into the calico envelope of her skirt between her knees.

The attraction between them was mighty, and that was no good. If Sam and Helen felt they had to marry, then Sam, who had not yet joined the church, would be separate from his people—although not excommunicated or shunned.

Helen, after all, had not worked from sunrise to sunset, indoors and out, on a farm for her entire life; she hadn't been quilting since she was seven; she had no idea how to whip up, without sweating, a vat of silken mashed potatoes for fifty Amishmen raising a barn; she couldn't bake twenty pies on a Friday afternoon for church on Sunday, scrub her entire house from top to bottom on Saturday, serve ten or fifteen families their dinner at Sunday noon, and have everything entirely back to normal by two-thirty the same day. Helen knew no Pennsylvania Dutch. Shirts, trousers, and dresses did not stream from her sewing machine on winter evenings. Had Helen tried to put in a garden, she would have had to lay her rows out with rulers and plant her seeds in flawless straight lines as a way to know what was coming up. Helen didn't know the order in which to hand out the clothes. Her faith was an adaptation of sentiments expressed on wall posters of kittens.

Helen, not having grown up on a farm, wouldn't become Amish and live the Amish way. "And give up nursing and my new blue Toyota?" she asked, incredulous. And even if she were willing, the chances of her succeeding weren't good. Some few have tried to adopt the Amish way; very, very few have succeeded.

So Sam would have to compromise his way of life; he would give up having it intertwined with that of his family. He would not be at home for dinners, harvests, sings, snacks, frolics; he would not be there for births or weddings or family celebrations. He would not be asleep on just the other side of the wall when his mother died in her sleep.

Sam's mother did not make light of the friendship;

she looked straight at Helen and said, "I suppose you'll take Sam away from us," and later Helen would giggle and say to me, "She's so silly to think that. I'm not going to hurt anybody," and she'd go back to embroidering initials on a handkerchief for Sam and planning picnics for the two of them. By then they were seeing each other, one excuse or another, almost every day of the week.

Sam's mother had put her life into raising her children Amish. Everything in Sam's upbringing, like every other child's upbringing, was designed to protect against the temptations of Helen.

From birth to five he would have lived, like every child, in his family's lap. Walk through any Amish farmyard and toddlers are underfoot as much as chickens. Should one be frightened by a sunflower that trembles like a temperamental dragon when the wind gusts, should one step barefoot on a twig, should one's eyes fill with tears, then up one is scooped into the cradle of Amish arms. One gets a soft ride then from here to there, while one's brother or sister or mother or father moves from flower bed to grape bower, from milking stool to hay loft. In the early years, you could say, a child is secured to the culture by abundant affection and belonging.

By the time they are five, children know they are not just wanted in the family; they learn they are needed and are valuable: They are depended upon to feed chickens, set the table, fold clothes, and run small errands for the bigger people in the family. In that year also, like children on the outside, they arm themselves with clean clothes and lunch pails; they assemble older sisters and brothers in phalanxes about them and make the first of eight years of morning marches to the schoolhouse.

If you ever drive through Amish country, you'll pass the white one-room schoolhouses where the children get their formal education. The schoolyards are carved square out of the cornfields; they are fenced and include two outhouses, a softball field, two swings, a pump, a teeter-totter, and the schoolhouse, inside of which the children learn the basic skills; reading, writing, geography, spelling, and arithmetic. They're not much on science, literature, politics, history, or other such material. Learning is by rote, repetition is the main activity; discussion and ratiocination are left for the English. The disciplines of being Amish are once again repeated; the ways of the outside world are neglected.

Helen asked me to help her once at an inspection for lice on the heads of children at one schoolhouse.

The stragglers were just slipping in the door when we pulled into the schoolyard. We followed and were welcomed by the teacher, Anna Mae, an eighteen-year-old Amish girl, satisfactorily equipped for her teaching responsibility by having completed—some years ago—an eighth-grade education in an Amish one-room schoolhouse.

Light poured in through double hung windows that lined either side of the classroom. The casements were pine, cleanly sanded and glossily finished. Displayed on the walls in geometric proportions was the students' work. Each student had colored in the mimeographed outline of an autumn leaf. Each child had applied the same combination of colors—brown stem, gold veins, orange palms tinged with scarlet. Each leaf had apparently drifted to the same October pond, for each one floated on the same crayoned field of blue. Some children did press hard—revealing, perhaps, a regrettable tendency to showiness—but none went out of the lines. On the far wall of the room, again symmetrically arranged, more school papers: each child's name had been drawn by the teacher in pudgy script and colored in by the student.

At the back of the room, at head's height, was a pine plank with dowels set in it. Black jackets topped by flat-brimmed straw hats hung along the length of it. Two shelves, also of pine, also glossily finished, held, in military order, girls' bonnets of black and navy blue, not a ribbon dangling. Another shelf held one straight stack of identical blue binders and one straight stack of identical textbooks. Beneath the shelves were benches. On them were seated three pairs of Amish parents all looking patiently, passively ahead.

The desks, each with its hardwood fold-up top, each with its narrow pencil trench, each with its wrought-iron legs, were arranged in six neat rows, eighth-grade boys to the rear of the class, first-grade girls—in full black smocks and uncovered knots of hair—to the front. Running across the front of the room, reminding the students not so much of the superiority of the teacher as of her authority, was a low dais. On it was positioned teacher's desk, neatly kept, with sharpened pencils, small stacks of student work, a tray of accepted texts, attendance and grade books.

At the back of the room, a folding table had been erected for Helen and me to work at. We sat down—I was assigned to keep the records of who had nothing, who had nits, and who had lice—and prepared to begin our inspection of heads. The three women at the back of the room stood up and came over to help. One, an older woman, smiled contentedly and patted her belly while she waited; the second, dour and drawn, scuttled restlessly back and forth behind our table. The third, a mound of woman hood built on pedestal legs, stood next to us and made wisecracks to the children as we went along. She had a toddler with her and he, with the natural arrogance of a loved child, crawled from scholar's bench to scholar's bench, assuming that each would move over and give him paper and crayon—and each one did.

Of the thirty-six children on the roll call, three quarters were named Stoltzfus (Stoltzfus being by far and away the most common name among the Amish); there were three Riehls and one Lantz child only. A mother asked if we could start with the girls so that the parents could leave sooner. I didn't understand the request because I didn't have the faintest idea why we had three sets of parents for helpers when we were just going to finger the children's hair.

Someone announced that the eighth-grade girls should let down their hair.

Twelve-year-old Ruth Stoltzfus raised her hands to the knot at the back of her head, pulled out a dozen pins, lifted and loosened her hair, which then billowed full and thick. As she walked to the back of the room, her head lowered and her eyes to the floor, her blond hair rippled down the slope of her back and gently stroked the inside curve of her waist. Ruth vaguely understood the power her hair had to seduce. She knew very well that the allure was not fitting for an Amish girl.

Helen took the strands of Ruth's hair and, not noticing the torment she stirred, let them fall through her fingers. A couple of the older boys sitting at the back the room were confused by an interest they hadn't felt before. Their minds left equations and field rows and drifted vaguely toward... what? They snuck glances at the falling hair. Ruth Stoltzfus blushed and kept her lashes lowered to her cheeks.

While Ruth sat with Helen, the rest of the students began work. The older boys taking the lead, they finally managed to get their math books open to the proper page, to get paper out and problems copied. Anna Mae called the first- and second-grade girls to the dais for a drill. They stood facing her and the blackboard. Anna Mae shuffled through flash cards of vowels, giving each child in turn a chance to get the answer right. A heavy redheaded girl, three times the size of her tidy, tiny peers, missed more than the others because she had to keep tugging at loose elastic in her panties with one hand and still remember to raise the other to show she knew the answer. Some horrendous conditions—loose elastic in a schoolgirl's panties, for example—cross all cultures.

While we worked, they worked. The idea was not to outperform the other fellow. I saw no signs of gold stars or of star students. As much as possible, the students were kept even in their learning; they worked together and helped each other. They took turns. They waited. In the classroom and schoolyard they learned, as much as anything, the ways of friends thye could expect to work with for the rest of their lives.

By this time, the corner of the room where the older girls were sitting was cascading with girls' hair, all of it floating with irregular freedom all of it needing to be chased back into its own tight little bun.

The three mothers fell upon the heads with combs unsheathed—three vigilant mothers to restore symmetry and discipline. Each head was wetted down and combed flat, each had its precision part restored. Twists of hair were knit once again tightly over ears and long strands were stretched straight out in parallel lines and whipped evenly into rope. Then, each rope, now indistinguishable from that on the next head, was tightly would, containing itself, well secured by bobby pins. Only when all heads were smooth, slick as kitchen countertops, could the mothers relax, go to their husbands, and ask to have the buggies brought around.

By recess time, we had finished the heads of all the boys and girls. For the record, the count was four heads with lice, three with nits, and the rest were clean. Helen and the parents gathered to work out prevention and treatment plans—who would tell Daniel's parents for example, and would we maybe be driving our car that way because by buggy it was a long way around? While we talked, the children made a circle about us, watching and studying. Until we drove away, the older girls hugged younger children to them, protecting them while they observed us.

The children, then, stay sequestered in their home and neighborhood schoolhouse until they are twelve.

After twelve there is an apprentice adulthood. Boys start working full days in the fields with their fathers or they work out as hired boys on neighboring farms. Girls work alongside their mothers or they, too, work in the fields or they may work at cleaning house for other families, either English or Amish. Officially, their lives remain governed by their parents. They do what they are told, go where they are allowed, receive what they are given. They are silently guided by the sameness of the lives around them and by the constant reminders that they are needed, wanted, cared for, understood, and protected. These conditions seem to be good ones. The young people seem strong and vital.

Then come the treacherous years: those between the time that children turn sixteen and the time that they are baptized and get married. Their freedom, their being set out without tethers, is considered necessary because only then will they be able to make a genuine choice about whether they will ask to be baptized and to join the church. It's the roaming, of course, that's so hazardous. Exposure to fast cars and true love can uproot in the young even those values that are most deeply, regularly, and rigorously implanted.

"Running around" the Amish call it.

I remember once, not too long after I moved to Lancaster, when I still felt that I should keep my voice down all the time because it seemed like I was living in a massive, dirt-floored, unceilinged church. It was Sunday night, a time of special modesty and subduing of the earthly passions. It was about 3:30 A.M., I had just finished a delivery, and the sky was exploding with rain, charging the earth with thunder and lightning. The best of all nights of the year to be home snug in one's bed, a Bible on the bedstand.

As I drove home, I saw more buggies per square mile of road than I had ever seen in a day. One after another buggies came toward me, their high-stepping horses in flashy poses against the electric sheets that flashed across the wet, black sky. Each buggy contained a young couple totally alone, idling, for heaven's sake, way deep into the morning hours, doing who knows what. They seemed not to be paying any attention to social order then, and it was only one short hour before milking time.

I couldn't believe my eyes. These young people—the same young people who but a few years before had been hanging on the schoolyard fences waving in innocent glee at passersby—were out carousing on a Sunday night, irrespective of all that's holy. This was a tragedy, one more in a long line of modern tragedies. Sex-indulgent, drug-distorted, authority-flaunting, punk-rock America had made its final, irreverent incursion—it had kidnapped the gentle youth of Lancaster County. I was sure I was seeing the last generation of Amish.

But no. As it turns out, they weren't following mainstream youth into garish, pointy-toed anarchy. They were merely "running around." "Running around" means that on her sixteenth birthday, a girl makes a new dress, no different from all the others she has ever worn except for some decorative stitches on the sleeve cuffs, and on Sunday night, she joins a "gang" at a sing in somebody's barn.

That's what I saw that night. A bunch of young people who'd been out all night singing. Singing, an activity different than, say, snorting or shooting up.

I later learned that the gangs— who call themselves things like "Antiques," "Sparkies," and "Luckies"—are, in fact, worldly to different degrees. Some do stick to singing and do keep the Amish code, but others experiment more freely. Boys might wear wristwatches, drink beer, and—in extreme and serious cases—find musicians with plug-in electric guitars.

It's when such musicians play in a barn just down the road from the preacher's house that the older generation—minister, bishops, and fathers in black frock coats—gather the young and remind them of the order to be kept in one's father's barn.

Girls rarely get pregnant before they are married in Lancaster County. And that's even though they take trips to the Jersey Shore, to the beaches at Sarasota, and to Niagara Falls. (You can hardly get out of an Amish bedroom without gazing on a velvet painting of Niagara Falls.) So far from home the girls join the boys for bike rides along beaches and through parks at sunrise.

Some boys buy cars, which they keep in neighboring towns, available for nighttime runs. Helen's Sam had been one of these: in fact, he'd been off to the West, where he'd worked on a ranch for six months. Others, making the same exploration of the world, get ensnared in situations they understand little; they do, in fact, do drugs. The life of a church elder includes trailing off to different parts of the country to gather stray youth.

Besides those young people who wander off for adventure, some of the youth—propelled by inborn curiosity, insatiable intelligence, a desire for greater freedom, a longing for a non-Amish career or for another faith—choose to leave the community. They elect to go on to school; they elect to believe things other than their families believe.

All in all, a little over 20 percent of the children born to Amish parents do not remain Amish.

It finally happened, of course, that Helen and Sam —probably excited from having been caught in a summer thunderstorm—got to kissing one another during the buggy ride back home. Helen had me believing that it started when they were clip-clopping through a covered bridge, that there had been snow and black-toothed trees before they entered, and pink blossomed boughs as they exited.

Apparently Sam started thinking seriously about

courting Helen, but the more he got to feeling like it, the harder it got. He spent a lot of time with a close friend and his wife in those days. They were getting ready to move to their own farm in another county. Sam decided to go with them and be their hired man for a year.

Helen insisted that the only thing in life for her was nursing. It had always been nursing, she said.

XX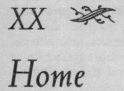

Home

Richie and I had been living in the rented house with the four-plant tobacco crop for two years when he began to search for land to build a house on. He studied plots in the clerk's office, on maps, and from the cockpit of a small plane, and eventually found a southward-facing slope with a copse of trees. He calculated that the land would be within driving radius of my patients and determined that it could not be used for farming. Richie refused to build on land that an Amish farmer could make good use of.

Standing on the slope, we looked over a ribbon of a tossing green cornfield, to a tobacco plot dotted with fat-leafed bouquets and, beyond that, to an effervescent band of alfalfa. A pasture lay to the east. At a neighborly distance was a farmhouse, two barns, a silo, and a windmill. Beyond them, more fields lapped into the distance, interrupted only by an occasional farmhouse. We could see miles across the gentle valley to the hills.

An Amishman, the one who followed his team of

horses across the flow of fields below the woods, allowed us to buy this piece of his land.

Richie meant to make the basic design of the house himself. He stuffed rolls and rolls of flimsy paper under his arm and disappeared into the back room, and hours, or days, later he'd come out with pencil drawings of houses with turrets and houses with sunken bathtubs and houses with circular staircases. Timidly, I'd talk to him about them, offering praise and suggestions here and there. Richie'd go back and erase things and make more drawings. He flew out to California to see some houses he'd read about. He made more drawings. He made them into a series of blueprints.

I kept quiet.

One night, after he'd spent months and months in the back bedroom drawing and redrawing on the flimsy paper, Richie woke up, jumped out of bed, went to his drawing board, and destroyed everything. The drawings were wrong, he said. He had been designing houses for someplace else. He had to go back to the beginning and make a house for Amish country.

The Amishman does not impose himself on his piece of land because, in a fundamental way, he does not really own it, not the way English own property. Instead, he considers himself its steward. It is his privilege to live on it; the land is in his trust during his lifetime. He is so serious about being a faithful steward that he nurtures his earth, he brings forth the harvest of its own disposing, he tends the land until it glows with contentment. It's just his work, his assignment, he would say, coming from Genesis. He, the Amishman, follows God's design; he is supposed to "replenish the earth, and subdue it: and have dominion over the fish of the sea, and over the fowl of the air, and over every living thing that moveth upon the earth." (Genesis 1:28) And so he believes he does.

But to me, he doesn't "have dominion." Dominion means dominating; running the thing, being the king. Americans, crashing through the forests, tilling the plants to dust, fishing the seas empty, assumed that the earth was their dominion; that it was theirs to do with just as they pleased.

The Amishman follows the earth; it tells him when to rise and when to sleep; it tells him what he can and can't plant and when. The Amishman treats the land sensitively—he nourishes it with horse and cow manure; he treads on it lightly—with teams of animals instead of machinery that packs it down. He works it often by hand. The Amishman's fields flourish because he pays close attention to them, because he is sensitive to the earth, because he lets it guide him.

I don't know how many times he crosses his rows in a year or in a lifetime, but each time he crosses he pays attention. When he and his horses pull a blade over the field, he bends from the waist to see the dirt being sliced. He learns from being the earth's bedfellow in all seasons. Because he is sensitive to the earth, it is abundant and beautiful.

In the same way that an Amishman discovers the best in his land and helps it produce, Richie found the house in himself, from the people who were our neighbors and from the land around us.

A crew of ten Amishmen built the passive solar, post-and-beam house Richie finally designed. The Amish contractor had built twenty-odd barns or so and knew post-and-beam barns better than anyone in the country; he didn't have so much experience with houses, but he allowed he'd "just tell the boys it's a house and not a barn."

The roof line follows the slope of the hill and the shape of the woods around it. Looking up at it from the road below, the house seems like it belongs, like it settled in centuries ago. From Reuben's farm, it's barely noticeable—especially now, as the trees grow up in front of it. We keep our lamps turned from the windows, so that the Amish darkness is not disturbed by our show of electricity.

The living room, which takes its shape from an octagonal framework of oak beams, spreads in a low apron out toward the rows of corn and into the woods. Since the room is bounded floor to ceiling on four sides by oak-framed glass, the sun and light move almost freely in it as they do beyond its windows. At the autumn equinox, the sun rises precisely at the easternmost window and sets at the westernmost. The ceiling is webbed by the golden oak beams, which radiate out from a massive stone column. Pine planks form the ceiling proper. In the center of the house we have a two-story atrium, which gives light to the underground portions of the house and makes my indoor plants content. The house stays cool in the summer and we don't start the coal stove until late in October.

The rooms have a unique shape—shapes so distinct that I believe they are more natural to Richie than square rooms.

Each room is white, each has a pine ceiling, each has been bisected at angles with oak beams. Windows reflect in windows. Angled beams, posts and dowels cast and pass one over the other triangular shadows, pentagonal shadows, square shadows, and shadows of leaves. The house lets in mist and sun, dusty colors from the plowed fields; snow laces the skylights, lightning often freezes for an instant on the white walls.

The house's structure—those muscular oak beams—give me protection and distance from the demands of practice. Each time I come in, I feel like I am entering a silent cave with a broad opening facing only the fields and forests.

It's right for Richie and me here. Neither of us cares much for the city. When he gets back from a trip (Richie's now flying 727's, and I think no other man could imagine how happy he is to be doing it), he works on the house. Slowly he is completing the finishing work upstairs; this last summer he labored at a rock wall. For myself, I put in a garden, put up green tomato mincemeat and the like; I cook, sew some, decorate. I go to quiltings and Tupperware parties with my Amish neighbors. We both play with the dogs and when they have puppies I am, naturally, a wreck for weeks.

Sometimes we'll take off on short romantic interludes: once Richie kidnapped me for a day—having worked out an arrangement with my back-up doctor to cover for me—and took me to New Orleans for a "proper creole dinner." Sometimes we'll go to Dallas to roust with Richie's old friends or we'll meet in New York for brunch. The truth is, though, for both of us, the excitement crests not when we're there but when we see the first horse and buggy on the roads leading toward home.

I can't imagine not being married to Richie. I believe it's the same for him. I suppose it was settled that day when I came out here to practice five years ago. I acceded not only to whatever force it was that put me here, but also, a little bit, to the idea that there are things in life that must be and that the only wise action is to accept them.

As our marriage has grown, I suppose both of us came to accept that it simply is. We are fortunate, I suppose, in that both of us have work that means so much to us; it makes it natural to respect and support the other's work.

Richie has never let me down, never complained about my work—as disruptive to our daily lives as it is. He'll have to get up at four to get to a flight and, without fail, that's the night the phone will ring all night long. He doesn't say anything or show annoyance—he'll either roll over and go right back to sleep or stay semi-awake and follow the unfoldings.

He has a record of heroic efforts: for example, he's rescued me from snowbanks at three in the morning, and once, by means unknown to me yet, he found me at an obscure intersection in order to tell me that my radio had broken down and a call had come in for a delivery.

One night I was finishing one delivery when the call came in for another. Since I was near home, I decided to stop there and return the father's call. As I walked in the door—it must have been two-thirty or three in the morning—I saw Richie, standing in his pajama bottoms in the middle of the kitchen. "Uh, gosh, Aaron," he was saying, "I don't know much more about these things than you do, but if you think it would help, I'd be glad to come over."

XXI

Leah

Johnny, Leah's husband, called about four in the morning. He thought maybe I should come right over, so I went. Leah and Johnny were very important to me.

I met Leah the first summer I was here. Elizabeth, a new patient, had invited me to her house to make tomato soup. Shades of Nana's kitchen. I took the road through the corn rows to her yard and traipsed contentedly through her garden. I remember the pole beans were head high. Hanging from the grape arbor were bunches of dusky purple grapes. I ducked the morning laundry and turned into the washhouse-canning house.

Young Rebecca was pumping water into a slate basin piled with red and golden tomatoes. Lizzie was just coming in with bundles of yellow onions, each one tied by twine. Anna, just six and equal to errands only, was standing around with her hands on her hips waiting for a new order. Over the sink—where we would be rinsing and cutting celery, onions, green peppers, and parsley—was an open window, so that as we worked the wind would blow on us and we could smell grapes all at the same time.

By the time I got there, two huge blue-and-white speckled pots were bubbling on the stove. One held the first batch of tomatoes.

Leah, probably twenty years old at the time, was there with her mother. She was the shyest thing I'd ever seen, shoulders bent down and her arms folded over her stomach. Amish women often have their arms folded over their stomachs, but Leah made it look as if she were set on sinking into her own pelvis and disappearing. She wore glasses with dark heavy rims, her skin was pale—probably from having her head sunk down into her chest all the time—and she didn't speak. Her mother spoke for her. "Leah will help with the cutting," she would say and push Leah in the direction of the knife. "Leah's not really quite strong enough to put the vegetables through the grinder." I was sorely tempted to lose respect for Leah, but I thought I should give her a chance. Pushy mothers are pushy mothers, after all. So I tried to ask her questions to bring her out, but if she did answer at all, she tended to answer inappropriately. I concluded the girl was retarded.

Only one thing was wrong with my theory, and looking back, I probably skimmed right over it.

When we really got the tomato soup operation started, every station in the summer kitchen was being worked by a girl in a bright skirt, her fingers marching smartly from tomato to tomato. I was at the slicing table with Leah. We were busily coring and cutting and dropping the sections into a massive pot when along came Anna, and quick as a green frog, she jumped up on the table, squatted down in the mushroom made by her skirt, grinned at us, stuck her arms into the pot right up to her armpits, and began to squeeze tomatoes. She squeezed a few, they burped and belched and oozed from between her fingers, and she looked up at me and Leah and grinned like she was getting away with murder. She wasn't—she was supposed to be squooshing tomatoes—but it wasn't lost on her that it was a lark, squatting on the table with everyone around her while she mashed tomatoes with her hands.

She laughed. She pulled her red-stained arms up out of the pot, turned to me, made her hands into claws, her mouth into a curl, her voice into the sound of a vicious dog, and started moving across the table, as if she were the enraged beast and I the helpless lamb.

I shrieked, which made her adore me, and then back she went to squeezing tomatoes.

Leah seemed to forget herself for a moment. Her shoulders straightened, her eyes lit up, she reached down into the pot of tomato soup herself, and while Anna's back was turned, she dipped three fingers of each hand into the pot, drew them down across her face as if to look like a savage avenging a kidnapped child, tapped Anna on the shoulder. Anna turned round, and Leah hissed, a dry, steamy and sharp-toothed hiss. Anna nearly jumped into the pot with fright and almost immediately begged, "Do it again." Leah did, and Anna batted a tomato claw at her, and I thought the two of them were going to get down on the floor and start rolling around like lion clubs. Suddenly I saw Leah's mother, her mouth looking like it had just been dusted with lye. She said, "What's going on over there girls?" Apparently Leah didn't hear. Her mother looked like she was headed toward us, so I reached over and tugged at Leah's apron. She looked up quickly and froze. I nodded in the direction of her mother, mimed as if to wipe my face, and Leah got the idea. By the time her mother came over for her deportment inspection, Leah had sunk right back down into her doleful, ashamed way.

After that Leah disappeared back into the shadows; except when she left she looked straight at me and smiled.

I heard from Elizabeth that Leah got married that November. Hard to imagine how that happened, but, then, I don't always see these things. Maybe the fellow had seen her imitation of the savage avenger. Maybe the flicker came out when the girl was away from her mother's granite presence.

Come March, when I get my first batch of pregnancies from last year's November matches, in comes Leah. She and Johnny—having lived, like all Amish brides and grooms, at her parents' house for several months—had just moved into their own house and they were abuzz with excitement.

Leah wasn't as hunkered over as she had been, and her eyes glowed even though she didn't lift her face too much, and she still couldn't fit two words together without furrowing her brow, and when I asked her questions she got the answers wrong. But she was wondrous when I confirmed for her that she was pregnant—even though now she was five months along, even though her tummy was firm and plump as a watermelon, even though the baby was bouncing around inside on a pogo stick. "Why," she said, mumbling, "why, Penny, I didn't think it could happen while we were still living with Mom and Dad."

I explained, but I wasn't sure at all that she was

following. Still, she went to her baby classes. She wrote down questions and handed the list to me when she came in for her checkups, and I'd answer the questions while Johnny stood there and listened and acknowledged the answers. Leah stared at me while I talked, as if fascinated, but I had no confidence at all that she understood.

She and Johnny never missed an appointment; they were never arrogant (in fact, they were properly awestruck by the whole business), and they seemed very respectful and loving of one another. They were courteous to me.

About a week before the baby was due Johnny called and said he wondered if I might stop by, that Leah seemed to be having some pains. I asked him some questions—more to get him warmed up to the real thing than anything; I was almost a hundred percent sure the baby wasn't ready to go, but I told him I'd be by.

Sure enough, all she had were warm-up cramps and they'd disappeared totally by the time I arrived. I sat for a while, trying to help them get more comfortable, and then pretty soon Johnny asked if I might be able to do something for Leah, as long as I was there. Leah didn't hear real well, he said, and they thought that with the baby coming it might help some if she had her ears cleaned out. He'd heard of somebody who had that done and it improved his hearing quite a lot and, well, even if it only helped some Leah would be able to hear the baby crying better.

I said sure—the afternoon was just dawdling by anyway—and cleaned out her ears, getting out a record amount of wax, and went on my way.

The next week the three of us had a good delivery. No, it was a great delivery. Under Johnny's care, Leah was blooming, and the two of them gamboled through the birth, hugging each other and kissing each other with their eyes all the time. They just oohed and aahed all over the place when little Eli was born, and when he cried, Leah's eyes filled with tears. She looked at Johnny and at me and whispered, "Listen to that sweet cry."

We talked after the baby was born. Leah chattered about this thing and that, made jokes about her mother, acute observations about our mutual friend Elizabeth, and some thoughtful comments about a book she'd been reading on how to take care of babies.

Leah had been virtually deaf. With her ears cleaned, with Johnny's care, with a new baby, she was a transformed person. She was lively and funny. She began to thank me and they both thanked me and then they thanked me again and again.

Nothing could stop Leah and Johnny after that. He'd go off and work at a cabinetmaker's shop during the day and then come home at night and do chores on the farm where they were living. She tried to make sure the baby was awake for him to see when he did have a few minutes at home. They were forever making themselves picnics and going on rides and dancing around in the kitchen.

Somewhere early on, Leah got an infection that raged like crimson fire across her breast. I had never seen such patience in a woman. The pain had to have been excruciating, but she knew it was best for her baby to nurse. She stayed with it. I was with her one afternoon for about two hours while she patiently worked with her baby, talking to him, letting him sleep, waking him again, prompting him to nurse at the swollen breast, never losing patience with him, never attacking herself. It was as if nothing could harm her joy now; she had her Johnny, her hearing, and her baby.

I would stop by whenever I was out their way. I would bring them small presents and they were always giving me jelly and homemade bread.

Leah had trouble getting pregnant the second time. I suggested she and Johnny move back in with Leah's mom (I think that's the night they put salt in my tea), but since they wouldn't follow that instruction I taught them about herbs and timing, and even then it took about a year and a half after they'd first started trying. I'm not sure who was more excited about the advent of the new baby—them or me. For the first time in my midwifery life, I was prepared to take up knitting again.

Johnny called at four one morning. I'd just seen Leah a week before and everything was fine, and, in fact, Richie and I had been over to their house for a snack the night before. We had been teasing them about names for the new baby; Richie kept suggesting names of old friends from Maine. Couldn't you name the baby "the Squire of Barker Ridge?" he said. "You know, I don't expect to have any children of my own and I just think the Squire ought to have somebody named after him. The Squire taught me to drink beer, you know."

I heard fear in Johnny's voice when he telephoned. "Is she bleeding?" I asked. "No," he said, "she's having cramps. Penny," he said, "please come right away."

Premature labor, I thought. "Tell her to stay off her feet," I said. "It's probably just premature labor. I'll be right over."

I sped to their house. Johnny was at the door of my

car with the flashlight before I came to a halt. "She's still having cramps," he said, "only they're stronger." He put his hand on my arm, forcing me to stop before we got inside. "We were wondering, Penny," he said, his hand getting heavy, "she can't feel the baby moving anymore."

Leah was in the bedroom lying down, just as she had been instructed. She was on her side, her head resting on the palm of one hand, her other hand clutching a pillow to her breast.

There was fear in her face. "Penny," she said, "Penny, please help us. I can't feel the baby anymore."

I use a device called a doptone for deliveries. The doptone, placed against the lower part of the mother's abdomen, picks up the sound of the placental blood rushing in and out of the cord and, over that, it drums out the sound of the fetal heart. It picks the sounds up and magnifies them, throws them against the wall in warm, reverberating, overhead arcs.

I put the doptone against Leah's tummy and the ceiling did not echo. We heard the rush and flow of the placental blood, but the baby's heart did not break in tropical waves from the room. There was no fetal heartbeat. I continued the examination, knowing already what was going on, not knowing at all what to say about it.

I keep my composure at deliveries; that's a rule. It's a necessity. Of course, things often happen that are powerfully moving, but I'm not being paid to indulge my sensitive nature.

Leah and Johnny's baby was dead. Leah was dilated to nine centimeters, and contractions were coming one right after the other. I had no idea how I would keep my composure.

I cleared my throat and looked at them. "I don't get a fetal heartbeat," I said, as simply as I possibly could. "Your baby isn't living." And then, without warning, for the first time in my career, I looked at my patients and, with my eyes, asked them to help me. I couldn't do it alone, and what's more, I had no wish to do it alone. I needed and wanted them to be with me.

As I gave way to them, the fear left their faces. I breathed deeply and let tears fill my eyes. I went on. "Your baby isn't living, but it's about to be born."

Now they looked at one another. They too began to cry. In a few minutes I said, "You can have the baby here or we can call the ambulance. What would you like to do?" I waited.

Finally Johnny spoke. "Is it any safer one way or the other?"

"No. There's no more danger than if this were a live birth. There is no reason we can't do it here."

We waited in the silent room for a long while. The stillness comforted us. Perhaps it made us belive that time was not passing; perhaps it made us believe that the next minutes and their sad issue would not come. Silence spreads far, it encompasses eternity. If we were part of eternity too, then we would not really lose the baby.

After a while Leah said, "What do you think, Johnny?"

He waited and answered, "Whichever way you think, Leah."

"I want Penny to give us our baby now," she said.

Johnny went out to my car for my bag while Leah and I talked. How long had it been since she felt life? She wasn't sure. She remembered that the baby had been scrambling yesterday morning when she was baking because she'd been thinking it must be a boy it was fighting and scrapping so much inside her.

After that, she said, the baby was quiet, and she just thought he'd worn himself out.

I was somewhat relieved. If the death was recent, the chances were better that the fetus might be all right to look at, but we had no assurance. When Johnny came in and we were getting Leah settled on the blue delivery sheets, I felt I had to warn them. "The baby might be deformed, you know."

"That's all right," he said, "we understand."

By now the labor pains were coming more and more quickly. Leah flushed, perspiration gathered on her upper lip and brow; she was lost to her contractions. The labor reassured me; I knew about labor, I understood it. I slipped with relief into the coaching ritual, began to believe again that everything was all right. I abandoned myself to the rhythm, began to think we were just delivering Leah and Johnny's baby, when—again and again—I'd slam up against the fact.

Needing a good push from her, knowing I would get it if I promised her something good, the way I always did, I went on to say, "Give me a good push and then you can see..." I stopped midsentence. I know Johnny and Leah heard the missing phrase as loudly as I did. The truth bruised us again.

Then abruptly, before we were ready at all, in one sleek move, the silver baby whooshed out.

It came so quickly, with so little warning. I caught her from instinct. Then, still moving from instinct, I reached for my suction. I pulled my hand back. I reached for a blanket to throw over the baby to keep it warm. I pulled my hand back. Was there nothing I could do? What about all those urgent, life-ensuring necessities? I let my hands down and let the child lay, one arm tucked under her chin, her legs loosely bent at the knees, her eyes closed. She was smooth-skinned, as if very finely made. I was riveted by the look of peace on her face. And profoundly confused by the umbilical cord knotted so tightly about her neck.

"It's a baby girl," I said. "The cord is wrapped around her neck."

I couldn't tell whether it was a sob or a moan from a contraction that broke out of Leah like a hand grasping for help. Anguish, perhaps, expressed by the cramp. The afterbirth came.

Birth usually feels like a steamy kitchen—similar to holiday preparations except that the smells are different. The smell of sweat is more acrid, there are some fetid odors, there is the smell and steam rising from blood. The air is thick, pungent, fertile. It is hard not to be reminded of fresh straw and night stars. There is near and heady promise.

As birth comes closer, the attendants gather around the bed. People who have never shaken hands intertwine their arms, touch their heads. Strangers breathe sympathetically for strangers, they massage, they stroke, praise, tease, cajole, whisper, wipe, instruct, hold, hug, discipline. Strangers give to strangers the best that they believe in, whole, stripped of wariness.

Because the outcome is never certain, the bond stays set until the baby is breathing, washed, wrapped, and sucking at its mother's breast.

This baby came in a streak of pallid light. The light from the lantern did not mist through the room. There was no fountain of fluid, gushing out. There was no wrestling with life, no contending, no grabbing it—as babies seem to grab—holding tightly to the progress they make through the passageway. No grabbing life by the fists. Just a sleek silver-dipped baby sliding out.

It lay on the bed while I worked. I kept looking down, surprised, disbelieving. At this moment I wasn't struck so much by grief as by confusion. The baby's body was magnetic; but as I said, it wasn't her death. It was the absence of life.

There should have been heat—I should have been working and massaging my life into hers. Usually I felt as if I was helping give life, but here I was unneeded; death managed for itself.

At the moment I wasn't sad. I just felt left out. We—father, mother, and midwife—were totally and completely irrelevant. Death dismissed us; the child had been tapped by another order, one with concerns we didn't know. At first I felt genuine respect. Death was sure, uncompromising. Then, curiously, I felt peace. The death was not my fault. The death was not the parents' fault. We didn't have a chance. The force that took this baby was impossibly, imponderably vast.

For a moment, I felt an exquisite freedom; light with relief. Death does not consult us. We had nothing to say. It was not our responsibility. And if this was true, perhaps we were not consulted on other things either.

I wrapped the baby in old soft flannel. I covered her and carried her to her parents. I wanted to hold her, caress her, and praise her. Maybe it was just the ritual, something in honor of what I missed or what I missed in her. I said nothing, however, not knowing what her parents would want. I carried her around the bed to them and showed her. I showed her face and body, where the cord was still around her neck. They began to stroke her ever so gently and to praise her. "She looks just like her brother, Eli, when he was born. . . . Look at her sweet eyes and tiny ears. . . . I am so sorry that she had to struggle."

I offered to wash the baby up and took her to the kitchen. I meant to squeeze golden shampoo on her head to freshen her, to dip her little head underneath the water, until all the soap ran away and only new baby smell stayed. But when I touched her skin, it began to fall away. Besides, I couldn't have washed her; the old flannel clung to her skin.

I was taking instructions at something new. Each time I tried to give the baby life, death slapped me down, death reminded me that I was intruding when I had no right, no business. The affair was not mine.

The baby's skin was fragile, as if it were determinedly melting into the soft web of the cotton fibers. The baby knew better than to let go of the closeness of the cloth; it was as if it had found itself at home, as if it were single-minded about becoming part of the things, part of the earth. Again I felt reproached; I backed off, embarrassed.

I wrapped the baby in a receiving blanket and gave her to her mother. Leah was crying again and so was Johnny. She studied the baby, talking to her through her tears, talking so softly and lightly that I could not make out her words. At the same time, she talked with me and Johnny about the funeral arrangements.

After a while I left them and packed my things. When I went back into the bedroom, Johnny was sitting silently on the edge of the bed with the baby nestled on his knees. He was rocking slowly back and forth. Leah was sort of propped up against him. Johnny chanted, "Oh, sweet little baby, little baby, oh." I went over and kneeled by Johnny's knee and he put his arm around me, and for the longest time he rocked me too.

I walked out of the house just as the sun was coming up and the November frost was glistening on brisk green sprouts of winter rye. I walked out to my car, stopping for a minute at the barn door to watch the Amishman at his milking. Lantern light filtered across the beams on the barn roof and sifted down below. About half the cows were down, the others shifted their weight and chewed hay. The farmer moved the milking lines from one cow to the next. He shuffled pails. A four-year-old girl—her green dress pulled over her knees, a babushka tied under her chin, hands folded patiently in her lap—sat waiting while her father milked.

I drove along the hand-patted roads. A lone buggy came toward me; its young driver raised his hand and waved. The mist began to blush. I passed Ebersol's pansies, planted in September for March sales. Their lavender, white, purple, and pink blossoms tossed in the morning breeze. I couldn't tell if it was springtime or winter. Birth and death kept mixing themselves up. Death took our baby. Death gave me something. My business was life; my life was concerned with giving life. I'd had no tolerance for death; it was a vicious thing. Now what was it? How did birth and death get themselves so intertwined?

Fortunately, life had to go on. I had to call on Leah's mother. I had to get the death certificate. I had house calls to make. I had phone calls to make. I had to get some groceries.

The sun had the sky now. Children skipped like clusters of rabbits along the side of the road—boys still in their summer straw-brimmed hats, girls' white coverings gleaming. Their red lunch pails bounced along beside them. I turned at the third lane on the right.

The farmhouse, an old stone Normandy, had taken on the uneven roll of the earth that it sat on. It looked as much a fit as an old man in his evening chair. The barns and outbuildings were freshly painted crisp yellow and the earth around them was gold, and even though it was November, marigolds were tumbling energetically through the front yard fence. The front door was thrown open. Leah's mother was cleaning.

She shut the door firmly after me, ordered me into the kitchen to sit down on the bench, and demanded to know if I was fine. Excuse the mess, she said (there was none), she was in the middle of cleaning. Didn't I agree that it was a beautiful day? How was Richard?

I didn't know if I was going to make it through this. I'd forgotten what a bossy woman she was.

I answered her questions in order:

"Yes."

"Don't think of it."

"Agreed."

"Fine."

Then I told her that the grandchild she'd been expecting had died. She was about to make some remark that would have put whatever it was I had to say to immediate rest. But then she realized the meaning of my words and she stopped being the boss. She stood there and looked at me, and then she lowered her eyes and her whole body sobered. Then she looked at me again.

"Is Leah all right?"

"Yes."

"When did it happen?"

I told her.

"Are you all right now?"

"Yes."

"Well, then," she said modestly, "I believe I'll go tell Amos to get the buggy ready."

"Yes," I said.

Carrying the death certificate, I went to the funeral home. It was one of the few the Amish use. I'd passed it on the road, but had never given it any attention. Now, when I drove up, it offended me. There was the big drive with the white columns and overhanging portico. There was the massive maple, its autumn leaves a little too prettily secured onto long graceful limbs. There was the "home" itself, a former mansion, no doubt, big and brick, with a porch that curved pretentiously around the front of the place. The porch floor was glassy with fresh gray paint and accented by a strip of just washed plastic lawn.

The last thing an Amishman does is to unnecessarily ornament or advertise himself. He does not confuse showiness with value. I could not imagine an Amishman at this funeral home; I wanted to go to a place that looked like an Amishman's cabinet shop, a place with a kitchen garden outside and linoleum inside.

Inside, of course, more funeral decor. The carpet with the spongy bounce to it, the perpetual sepulchral afternoon lighting, the heavy chandelier, the demonstration coffins with the shiny gold handles, the black, glassy-faced grand piano and blue flocked wallpaper.

The owner greeted me and, of course, asked solicitously how he might help. I told him my business. I was bringing the death certificate for Leah and Johnny's girl and finding out if there was anything else I might do for them. The owner looked like he might have been transferred from a funeral home in 1950s California. His face was cut with small wires of age and smoking; he was tan and his hair was thick and grooved from being combed back with stick-um.

He was not cordial. To the contrary, he was contemptuous, as if I myself had slaughtered the child. I didn't know why—maybe he treated everyone like this, maybe he had medieval prejudices against midwives—but it didn't make any difference. I just knew that in the old days I would have been not cordial right back; I would have batted him with a couple of insults so quick and so final he would have dropped on his phoney rubbery carpet and bounced three times before settling.

I didn't. I didn't have the faintest desire to counterattack. I just got out the death certificate and handed it to him quietly and said I needed to ask a couple of questions to complete it.

"This death certificate won't do," he said impatiently. Something was as wrong on the inside of the funeral parlor as it was on the outside. It made me sad to think of my Leah and Johnny having to do business with this facetious, intolerant man. Yet the people spoke so highly of him.

He pointed me toward a counter, told me to put the certificate down and he would show me how to fill one out properly. "If you're going to do this kind of work," he said, implying that I'd picked up midwifery in Lancaster County the way one picks up a job washing dishes in a Bronx restaurant, "you're going to know how to fill out a death certificate." He paused, glared at me, and snarled, "Unless you think you're God or something."

If anything would have got me going, it would have been that, but I still didn't have the slightest urge to counterattack. What I knew best that morning was that I was not God. What I knew best was that I was a humble player in some mighty business that was so awesome and so powerful that I had abandoned all pretense of understanding it, let alone running it. That serene baby guided me.

I said I didn't think I was God.

The owner must have been caught offguard by the humbleness in my voice, because his lacerating tone softened for a moment, then he went on. He began to flick at the details of the death certificate. "You must spell out the month, do not write it in numbers." He lit a cigarette. "Put the mother's full name here. You must put in the cause of death, even though the people are Amish and may not have an autopsy; the state won't have it any other way." He puffed and paced behind the counter. Obviously the poor man had long been whipped by the state bureaucrats; he paid daily for their petty insistence on the uniformity of death, their impatience with customs any different than those they found allowable. I suddenly felt sorry for him. "You must put in the cause of death or you'll never get rid of the certificate."

I asked some questions that Leah and Johnny had asked me that morning before they had a chance to talk to their families. Finally I said, "Don't they dress the baby themselves?"

The man began to change. He began to explain that with most deaths the Amish make the clothes themselves. And a woman will probably wear the white apron and cap that she was married in. "They are very respectful and loving toward their dead." He went on, eagerness building: "Would you like to see the coffin and then I could tell you about how we'll care for the baby when we go get him?"

I could tell he wanted me to see the coffin. So I went. He took me back and led me to the small pine box. It was as simply made as possible—no handles, no trimming. Clean cut wood, countersunk nails, dressed only in its gray stain. He opened the lid, and with the tips of his fingers, he very carefully, very gently, unfolded the soft white batiste lining its insides.

"We'll wrap the baby in a downy covering," he said. "We touch stillborns as little as possible. Their skin is fragile and we don't want to cause any damage. That is the idea with one so small; touch them as little as possible."

He talked about his craft with great integrity; he became animated, young, vigorous. The bureaucrats lost their hold on him; the cynicism that had gripped him slowly vanished. His meanness disintegrated. I began to admire him.

I realized that he tried as hard to be gentle and considerate in his work as I did in mine. He respected the Amish; no, it was something more than that—he too had been deeply influenced by them. We began to understand one another. We talked.

"How long have you been a midwife?" he said.

"Five years."

"How many babies have you delivered?"

"About a thousand."

"Have you lost many?" he asked.

"One," I answered. "This one."

He was pulled up short. "Then I guess I won't be telling you anything about your work," he said deferentially. "Let me know any time I can do something for you."

It wasn't until I got back to Leah and Johnny's that day that I'd figured out why the funeral director had been so rude to me in the first place. I think he was just like me. Actively, fervently, and feverishly does he loathe the quacks who—driven out of hospitals—peddle themselves to the nonlitigating Amish and casually take their money and their lives. He had no reason to think that I was not one of them, bouncing into his shop to toss him my careless errors. I was guilty until proven innocent in his eyes. And in this case, his was, I believe, the proper attitude.

I couldn't go directly home that night. I was too restless, too ungrounded. As if something wasn't finished. As if there was something waiting for me yet. I passed the time by driving along the fields and by the streams, waiting to understand, waiting for whatever it was inside of me to finish its groping and shifting.

I came inevitably to the cemetery where we would bury the baby Susan the next day.

Amish cemeteries have no formal entrance. Laid out behind a whitewashed post-and-slat fence—little more set out than a pasture or a cornfield—the cemetery takes its turn like any other piece of earth along the road, its rows of headstones continuing the rows of corn stubble next to it.

It was warm for a November night. The sky was clear and the moon gleamed, but there was no wind. I pulled the car over to the side of the road, got out, and walked into the small cemetery. The grass inside, less well tended than an Amish women keeps her lawn, lay comfortably rumpled under the headstones. No flowers, no debris from dried bouquets, no loose ribbons from flower arrangements chattered or flapped in the wind. It was safe here from pretense and I could consider the baby's death.

As each Amish person wears the same hat or bonnet as his or her neighbor, each Amish person's headstone is like the one next to it. Each has the same shape—rounded at the top—and the same height and width. Each is unadorned except by time and the weather. One planted in this yard fifty years ago had darkened with age and, during the same years, moss, the color of goldenrod, had spilled ever so slowly down its face and into the crevices made by the letters. Another, next to it and brand new, flashed back to the moon its bright white marble face. Next to these two was a series of stones of slate, their faces smooth or fissured or broken off. The rows lined up, not precisely, because the ground had not been rolled by heavy machinery, but in good order. Down the path between them, at irregular intervals, were footstones. There is no unnecessary space left between one grave and the next.

The inscriptions are no more individual than the stones. It is enough to enter a man's name, the date of his birth, and the date of his death; also the number of days he had lived altogether. For a woman, her husband's name is also given.

I made sure to see that no one was coming up the road, and then, for a moment, I lay down to see if I would fit between a headstone and footstone. It hadn't seemed quite long enough or wide enough, but it sufficed.

The Amish are born, do their work—as directed by their abilites—and die. Each one of them has value because each one is part of the life of the earth. For them, to be part of the earth is to be part of God's work. That is enough of an awesome thing. No one life counts more than another; each life is necessary to the whole. During his time on earth, each man is responsible for being a steward of the earth, of his own life, of his inheritance, and of his brotherhood. During his time on earth, each person works to maintain well the portion of life they have received. Others follow and do the same. Each tries to be good and kind as they do so.

I leaned on the fence slats and watched for a while across the road at a cow barn, silo, tobacco barn, and farmhouse with porch, dressed with its wiry strands of grapevines. A farmer, carrying a lantern and followed by his dog, strolled to his barn.

I had believed that I was alone, that I created all my weakness and all my failures; I believed that I had created all my successes. I thought I had to be invulnerable, that I would have to survive in the universe on the strength of my personality and my will. I advertised myself and I made myself tough—hoping, I think, that the universe would admit that for the first time in its history, some Penny had come along who could outsmart it.

But I was no contestant against death. This baby's death so disregarded me that I no longer considered myself self-sufficient. That would be absurd. Other forces—forces far too mighty for me to comprehend—held sway. I had been silly.

Neither was I a contestant against gentleness. The Amish people live decently and kindly. They love what is. I've watched them keep their gardens and their farms with delicacy and respect. I've seen them adore the weak equally with the strong. I've known them to give themselves away completely when the brotherhood needed it. I've come to love their way—

soft, clean, and so often joyful. I've discovered the strength they have that comes from depending on one another. I've discovered the peace they gain in knowing that none of us is alone. I've discovered the freedom that comes in taking a smaller place in the order of things. I shrink now before their understanding of time, generations, life, death, and, yes, God.

The next afternoon I watched black carriages arrive at the cemetery. Nothing is more somber than that uninterrupted line, paced by a walking horse.

In the morning, some of Leah and Johnny's family and friends had come and dug the small grave.

I shivered and waited as the buggies pulled in. There weren't many, as big funerals are not the custom for stillbirths. The buggies were arranged at the fence, rows of headstones were arranged at my feet, and now at the graveside a row of Amish men and Amish women stood wearing their black hats and capes. The coffin, looking like an abandoned cradle, sat separate and independent on a small table. The baby was white, pure white—finished in porcelain.

Her tiny lips were blue. The woman next to me turned and whispered, "It makes you want to put a blanket over her, doesn't it?"

I stood with my arms clamped around me for warmth. Still I shook from the cold.

The Amish began to pray and so did I. I did not pray in their way but I prayed. As we stood in silence with our eyes closed and our heads dropped, a huge dark and warm wing folded round me. Johnny's father pulled me inside his cape to keep me warm.

About the Authors

PENNY ARMSTRONG has delivered over 1,000 babies. She is licensed to practice midwifery in the United States and is currently practicing in Lancaster County, PA.

SHERYL FELDMAN received her bachelor's and master's degrees at the University of Washington. She has worked in various social agencies and has known Penny for thirteen years.